KETO AIR FRYER COOKBOOK FOR BEGINNERS

365 Tasty And Easy Ketogenic Recipes For Every Day Of The Year To Quickly Prepare With Your Air Fryer

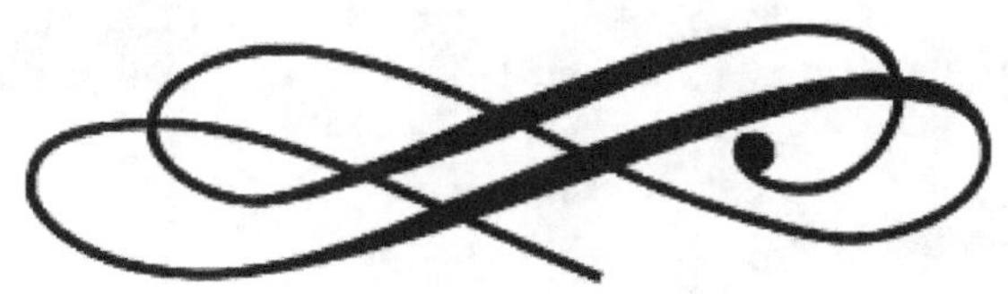

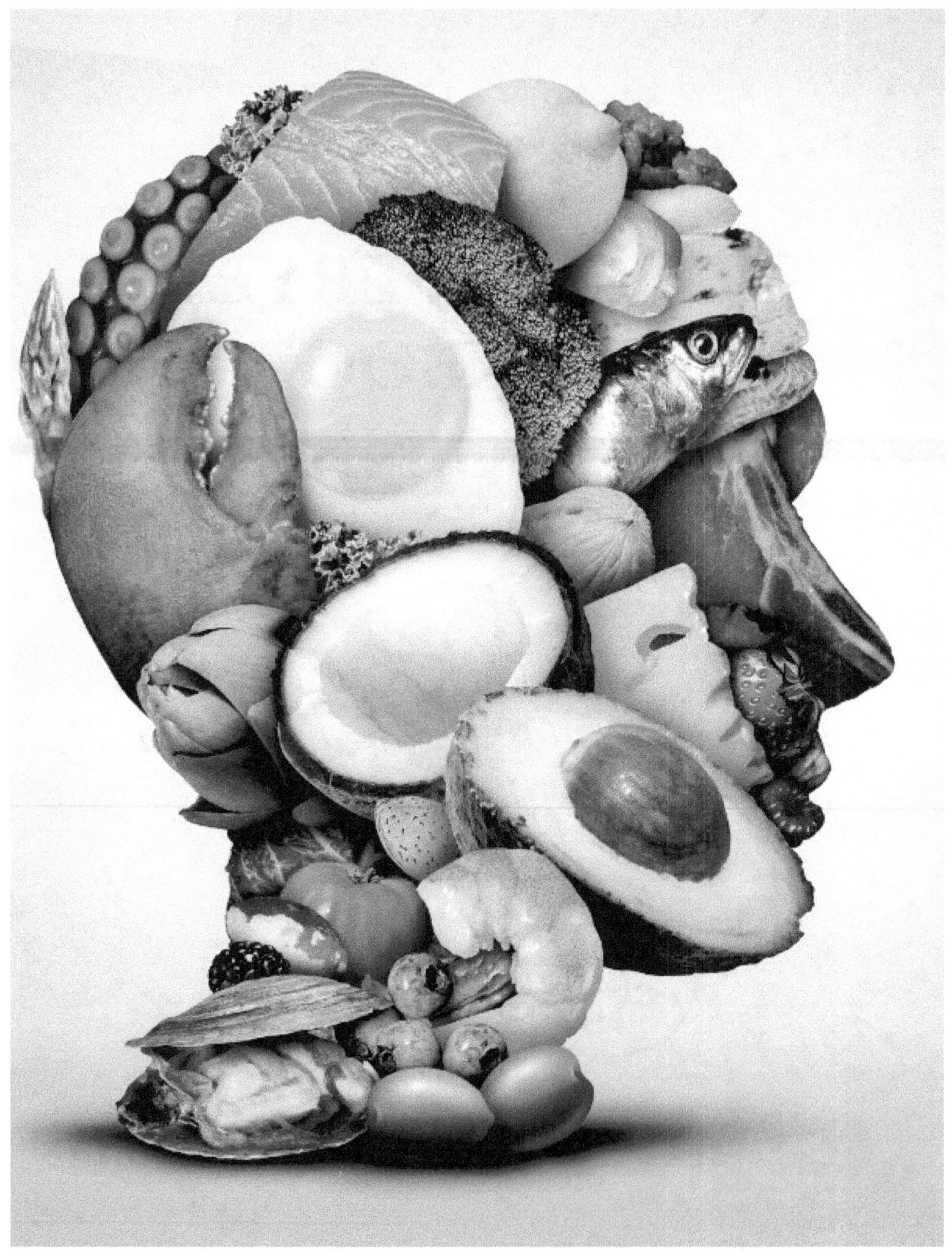

© Copyright 2020 - All rights reserved.

The content contained within this book may not be reproduced, duplicated or transmitted without direct written permission from the author or the publisher.

Under no circumstances will any blame or legal responsibility be held against the publisher, or author, for any damages, reparation, or monetary loss due to the information contained within this book. Either directly or indirectly.

Legal Notice:

This book is copyright protected. This book is only for personal use. You cannot amend, distribute, sell, use, quote or paraphrase any part, or the content within this book, without the consent of the author or publisher.

Disclaimer Notice:

Please note the information contained within this document is for educational and entertainment purposes only. All effort has been executed to present accurate, up to date, and reliable, complete information. No warranties of any kind are declared or implied. Readers acknowledge that the author is not engaging in the rendering of legal, financial, medical or professional advice. The content within this book has been derived from various sources. Please consult a licensed professional before attempting any techniques outlined in this book.

By reading this document, the reader agrees that under no circumstances is the author responsible for any losses, direct or indirect, which are incurred as a result of the use of information contained within this document, including, but not limited to, errors, omissions, or inaccuracies.

Table Of Contents

Introduction

The Air Fryer Toaster Oven has eight smart programs that give different cooking modes to the users, which are as follow:

Air Fry: using this program, to cook oil-free, crispy food, whether it's coated meat or fries, everything can be fried in its Air fryer basket.

Toast: the temp/time dial used to set the temperature and cooking time can be used to select the bread slices and their brownness when they need to be toasted using the Toast cooking program of the Instant Air Fryer toaster oven.

Bake: it is used to bake cakes, brownies, or bread in a quick time.

Broil: the broiler's settings provide direct top-down heat to crisp meat, melt cheese, and caramelizes the vegetables and fruits. It has the default highest temperature, which is 450 degrees F.

Roast: this cooking program is suitable for roasting meats and vegetables.

Slow Cooker: The Slow Cook program lets you adjust greater cooking time and lowest temperatures based on the requirements.

Reheat: using this mode, the users can warm up leftover food without overcooking the food.

Dehydrate: low-temperature heat is regulated to effectively remove moisture from foods, thus giving perfect crispy veggie chips, jerky, and dehydrated fruits.

For a longer usage or its span, always remember that the Instant Air Fryer Toaster Oven must be cleaned after every cooking session like any other cooking appliance. It is important to keep the inside of the oven germs free all the time. The food particles that are stuck at the base or on the oven's walls should be cleaned after every session using the following steps:

Unplug the Instant Air Fryer toaster oven and allow it to cool down completely. Keep the door open while it cools down. Remove all the trays, dripping pan, steel racks, and other accessories from inside the oven.

Place the removable parts of the oven in the dishwasher and wash them thoroughly. Once these accessories are washed, all of them dry out completely. Meanwhile, take a clean and slightly damp cloth to clean the inside of the oven.

Wipe all the internal walls of the oven using this cloth. Be gentle while you do the wiping. Use another cloth to clean the exterior of the appliance. Wipe off all the surfaces. Now that everything is clean, you can place the steel racks and dripping pan back to their position for the next cooking session.

For cleaning, do not immerse your appliance in the water directly. To clean the power plug, use a dry piece of cloth to remove the dirt.

Using this amazing air-fryer toaster oven can also help you prepare great taste foods savoring its great crunchy and juicy taste. Using an air-fryer is certainly going to help you to create better and healthier dishes.

Benefits of Using an Air Fryer
Reduced calories that can lead to weight gain and obesity
Reduced risk of high blood pressure
Reduced risk of heart disease and clogged arteries
Less chance of having a stroke or an aneurysm
Pros and Cons of the Air Fryer
Pros:
Much faster than regular frying alternatives
Versatile; can be used to bake, grill, roast, and more!
Easy to clean, thanks to the use of little oil
Obviously, air fryers are a much healthier alternative to oil frying. However, there are a few cons to consider if you are thinking about getting one of your very own:
Cons:
They are small and don't have a ton of room to cook items
Bulky and heavy in nature, even though capacity is rather small
Can get extremely hot, but not as dangerous as traditional oil fryers.

CHAPTER 1:

The Air Fryer

The air fryer is a nifty kitchen appliance that allows you to fry food at high temperatures using circulating hot air around the oil. This allows you to cook food evenly and faster compared to baking them in the oven. With this kitchen appliance, food is cooked with a delicious crispy layer, so you get the same effects of fried food without that greasy feel.

How Does It Work?

Air fryers are not only limited to frying food, but it also allows you to cook a wide assortment of food. Air fryers often come with the Rapid Air Technology that circulates extremely hot air of up to 4000F to cook food.

The air fryer comes with an exhaust fan that is located just above the cooking chamber. This provides an excellent airflow that is required to cook food, even those that are located at the bottom of the basket. The strong fan allows the food to get the same amount of temperature within the chamber. Moreover, it also comes with a cooling system to control the internal temperature so that the food does not burn while in the middle of cooking.

To cook food, place the food in the fryer basket and place the basket in the fryer and you can start cooking. Halfway through, give the basket a good shake in order to distribute the food evenly. The air fryer basket makes it easy to take the food out all at once, without the need to probe through the hot basket. It is as easy as that.

How to Use the Air Fryer

Using the air fryer is no rocket science—you can cook food easily even if you are a kitchen novice. It is important to take note that the air fryer comes with a cooking basket where you can place food. This makes it easier to handle your food while cooking.

First things first, make sure that you plug in the air fryer and allow it to preheat for 4 minutes. Make sure that the chamber is hot enough before putting the food so that the cooking process starts easily. It is always important to spray cooking oil to the fryer basket in order to avoid food from sticking to the basket. This will also make it easier for you to shake the food in the middle of your cooking time for even frying.

When placing the food in the fryer basket, make sure that you put space between each food so that the hot air can pass through and cook food evenly on all sides. You can use aluminum foil to separate large chunks of meat, for example, for even cooking.

When marinating the ingredients, make sure that you use dry spice rub as oil and sauces can cause smoke, as well as make cleaning of the air fryer more difficult. Should you need to put sauce or oil, do it at the end of cooking when you have taken out the food from the fryer. Never use a high temperature when cooking with fatty foods to avoid messes.

Frequently Asked Questions

It is easy to use the air fryer but if you are a first-time user, you must have a lot of questions about using the air fryer. Below are the frequently asked questions on how to use the air fryer.

1 – Can I cook different foods in the air fryer aside from fried foods?

The air fryer is not limited to cooking only fried foods. You can use it for cooking different types of foods like casseroles and even desserts.

2 – How much food do I need to put inside?

Different air fryers tend to have different capacities. If you are not sure how much you need to put in, look for the "max" mark and use it as a guide to filling the basket only to that part.

3 – Can I put in more ingredients while the food is being cooked?

Yes. Just open the air fryer so that you can add the ingredients that you want to put in. There is also no need to change the internal temperature as it can stabilize once you close the air fryer chamber.

4 – Can I put aluminum or baking paper at the bottom of the air fryer?

Yes. You can use both to line the base of the air fryer. However, make sure that you poke holes so that the hot air can pass through the material and cook food thoroughly.

5 – Do I really need to preheat my air fryer?

Preheating the air fryer can reduce the cooking time so you can save energy. Moreover, food comes out crispier. However, if you forgot to preheat, then that is still okay. You can still cook your food, but the quality is not as great as when you preheat the fryer. To preheat the air fryer, simply turn it to the temperature that is needed for cooking and set the timer for 5 minutes. Once the timer turns off, place your food in the basket and continue cooking.

CHAPTER 2:

Basic Rules of Ketogenic

How did most people who worked hard to lose a lot of weight end up getting it all back? Worse, why are some extra pounds usually tackled on, so folks end up weighing even more than before they began the whole diet process?

Many people believe they can eat, lose weight, and that's it! If the loss wasn't as significant as initially hoped, then they assume the same thing the medical establishment thinks; it's their (the dieter's) fault. They return to their pre-diet way of eating out of a sense of failure and eventually gain all that weight back plus a few extras!

Before you judge yourself or others harshly, though, there are several factors in this way of thinking. Our minds were trained to identify where we've gone wrong; we can move to a different way of eating and learning about the food we choose to consume.

So, what makes weight loss so difficult for millions? To answer this question, we need to look at the food industry and our dietary habits over the past decades, and how we have been taught to think about weight gain from the medical establishment and our governments. Over this period, there have been some changes that our manager how and what we eat daily that may contain some clues about what causes the obesity epidemic we are currently facing.

We'll continue with one of the biggest mistakes. The one that led to so much pain, feelings of shame, and embarrassment for the masses of people who worked hard to lose weight just to see each of those hard-lost pounds pile up. Sadly, it is a firm belief that the solution for obesity can be summed up in that essential phrase we all know so well; "Eat less–exercise more." Eat less, walk more. The commonly accepted idea is that for you to lose weight, the total calories consumed must be less than the calories burned. Thus, eat less –move more.

We're in the thinking camp that believes calories matter. However, if you're careful about your macronutrients, you'll automatically get the correct calorie count. They also accept that hormones are essential, so when designing recipes and meal plans for our Speed Keto system, they employ a balanced approach to ensuring insulin development is regulated.

When you are adopting a ketogenic diet, make sure to take care of the following food groups and combinations–they should not be included in your diet if you want to sustain the ketosis condition that you are bringing the body in.

Foods that are high in sugar, such as coffee, agave, tea, sports drinks, and maple syrup, must not be consumed. Sugar-sweetened foods should also be stopped.

Grains, along with grain-based foods, are prohibited. It covers granola, oats, grain, barley, pasta, and corn.

Some fruits will also be avoided due to their high amount of carbohydrates. Apples, oranges, and bananas are often considered at the top of the list when looking at fruit to avoid a ketogenic diet.

Tuber vegetables and food products made from these vegetables on the market are some of the items you can't eat. This would include carrots and yams, French fries, and potato chip packets.

While most people think that a ketogenic diet is restrictive, they will have to start eliminating many of the items they use to consume–the plan can still be rendered tasty and healthy. The goal here is to make sure you understand exactly what items you can include in your diet–and then use your cooking skills and imagination to develop ways to turn certain foods into healthy and balanced meals.

With a ketogenic diet, your consumption of carbs is relatively reduced. However, your intake of healthy fats is enhanced.

Types of items that come within the correct ranges to make them ideal for a ketogenic diet will have fish, such as oysters, mussels, octopus, squid, clams, and mussels.

Fish such as mackerel, tuna, and sardines.

Vegetables low in carbs, such as spinach, Brussels Sprouts, kale, cauliflower, and broccoli.

Cheese Poultry, including chicken and turkey.

Meat products, preferably grass-fed

Avocados Eggs, ideally omega-3-rich types,

Greek yogurt (unsweetened plain yogurt), Cottage cheese A variety of seeds, such as sesame seeds, pumpkin seeds, chia seeds, and linseeds.

Nuts, such as peanuts, macadamia nuts, pecan nuts, walnuts, Brazil nuts, cashews, and pistachio nuts

In addition to these food options, it is also important to note that, when cooking food, the three types of oil that you should use are avocado oil, coconut oil, and olive oil. Both three of these oils are considered to be rich in healthy fats and weak in unhealthy fats, and will not have a significant impact on your daily intake of carbohydrates.

Foods To Enjoy On The Ketogenic Diet

Different food types are listed here. These food ideas advocate for high-fat content while also labeling other foods and essential vitamins for the body to use.

Foods and Animal Products–Focus on grass-fed or pasture-raised fat cuts of meat and wild-caught fish, avoiding farmed pet foods and processed meats as much as possible. And don't forget the liver made meats!

Beef	Shellfish	Salmon
Hen	Chicken	Tuna
Chicken	Cat	Halibut
Eggs	Cow	Cod
Goat	Goat	Gelatin
Lamb	Lamb	Chicken fat
Pig	Pork	Coconut fat
Rabbit	Rabbit	Duck fat
Turkey	Turkey	Ghee
Venison	Venison	Lard

Tallow
MCT oil
Avocado oil
Macadamia oil
Extra virgin olive oil
Coconut butter
Coconut

Instead of root vegetables and other starchy veggies, you need to be vigilant about carbohydrates in the ketogenic diet, so stick to leafy greens and low-glycemic veggies. I've put avocados in this section because some of us may remember it as a vegetable even though it's a fruit.

Artichokes
Asparagus
Avocado
Broccoli
Bell peppers
Cauliflower
Cabbage
Celery
Cucumber
Lettuce
Kohlrabi
Radishes
Zucchini
Okra or ladies ' fingers
Seaweed
Tomatoes
Spinach
Watercress

Dairy Products– If you can handle dairy products, you can add full-fat, raw dairy products in your diet and unpasteurized. Keep in mind that some brands contain lots of sugar that could increase the carb content, so look out for nutrition labels and limit the intake of these items. When possible, go for the full-fat varieties as these are less likely to be used to substitute the fat with sugar.

Cottage cheese
Mozzarella cheese
Swiss cheese
Sour cream
Full-fat yogurt
Heavy cream

Herbs and Spices – Herbs and spices are an excellent way to flavor your foods while adding a moderate amount of calories or carbs.

Black pepper
Basil
Cinnamon
Cayenne
Cilantro
Chili powder
Cumin
Curry powder
Garam masala
Ginger
Nutmeg
Garlic
Oregano
Onion
Paprika
Parsley
Rosemary
Sea salt
Sage
Thyme
Turmeric
White pepper

Beverages: On the ketogenic diet, you can avoid all sweetened drinks, but there are certain drinks that you can still have.

Almond milk unsweetened
Bone broth
Cashew milk unsweetened
Coconut milk
Club soda
Coffee
Herbal tea
Mineral water
Seltzer water
Tea

CHAPTER 3:

January

Lunch

Mozzarella Tots

Preparation time: 12 minutes
Cooking time: 3 minutes
Servings: 5
Ingredients:

- 8 oz. mozzarella balls
- 1 egg
- ½ cup coconut flakes
- ½ cup almond flour
- 1 teaspoon thyme
- 1 teaspoon ground black pepper
- 1 teaspoon paprika

Directions:

1. Crack the egg in a bowl and whisk.
2. Combine the coconut flour with the thyme, ground black pepper, and paprika. Stir carefully.
3. Sprinkle Mozzarella balls with the coconut flakes.
4. Transfer the balls to the whisked egg mixture.
5. Coat in the almond flour mixture.
6. Put Mozzarella balls in the freezer for 5 minutes.
7. Meanwhile, preheat the air fryer to 400 F.
8. Put the frozen cheese balls in the preheated air fryer and cook them for 3 minutes.
9. Remove the cheese tots from the air fryer basket and chill them for 2 minutes.

Nutrition:
calories 166,
fat 12.8,
fiber 1.4,
carbs 2.8,
protein 9.5

Chicken Balls

Preparation time: 10 minutes
Cooking time: 8 minutes
Servings: 5
Ingredients:

- 8 oz. ground chicken
- 1 egg white
- 1 tablespoon dried parsley
- ½ teaspoon salt
- ½ teaspoon ground black pepper
- 2 tablespoon almond flour
- 1 tablespoon olive oil
- 1 teaspoon paprika

Directions:

1. Whisk the egg white and combine it with the ground chicken.
2. Sprinkle the chicken mixture with the dried parsley and salt.
3. Add ground black pepper and paprika.
4. Stir carefully using a spoon.
5. Using wet hands, make small balls from the ground chicken mixture.
6. Sprinkle each sausage ball with the almond flour.
7. Preheat the air fryer to 380 F.
8. Grease the air fryer basket tray with olive oil and place the sausage balls inside.
9. Cook for 8 minutes.
10. Turn halfway to crisp each side.
11. Serve hot.

Nutrition:
calories 180,
fat 11.8,
fiber 1.5,
carbs 2.9,
protein 16.3

Tofu Egg Scramble

Preparation time: 15 minutes
Cooking time: 20 minutes
Servings: 5
Ingredients:

- 10 oz tofu cheese
- 2 eggs
- 1 teaspoon chives
- 1 tablespoon apple cider vinegar
- ½ teaspoon salt
- 1 teaspoon ground white pepper
- ¼ teaspoon ground coriander

Directions:

1. Shred the tofu and sprinkle it with the apple cider vinegar, salt, ground white pepper, and ground coriander.
2. Mix and leave for 10 minutes to marinade.
3. Meanwhile, preheat the air fryer to 370 F.
4. Transfer the marinated tofu to the air fryer basket tray and cook for 13 minutes.
5. Meanwhile, crack the eggs in a bowl and whisk them.
6. When the tofu has cooked, pour the egg mixture in the shredded tofu cheese and stir with a spatula.
7. When the eggs start to firm place the air fryer basket tray in the air fryer and cook the dish for 7 minutes more.
8. Remove the cooked meal from the air fryer basket tray and serve.

Nutrition:
calories 109,
fat 6.7,
fiber 1.4,
carbs 2.9,
protein 11.2

Flax & Hemp Porridge

Preparation time: 10 minutes
Cooking time: 15 minutes
Servings: 3
Ingredients:

- 2 tablespoon flax seeds
- 4 tablespoon hemp seeds
- 1 tablespoon butter
- ¼ teaspoon salt
- 1 teaspoon stevia
- 7 tablespoon almond milk
- ½ teaspoon ground ginger

Directions:

1. Place the flax seeds and hemp seeds in the air fryer basket.
2. Sprinkle the seeds with salt and ground ginger.
3. Combine the almond milk and stevia together. Stir the liquid and pour it into the seed mixture.
4. Add butter.
5. Preheat the air fryer to 370 F and cook the hemp seed porridge for 15 minutes.
6. Stir carefully after 10 minutes of cooking.
7. Remove the hem porridge from the air fryer basket tray and chill it for 3 minutes.
8. Transfer the porridge into serving bowls.

Nutrition:
calories 196,
fat 18.2,
fiber 2.4,
carbs 4.2,
protein 5.1

Creamy Bacon Eggs

Preparation time: 10 minutes
Cooking time: 10 minutes
Servings: 4
Ingredients:

- 6 oz. bacon - 4 eggs
- 5 tablespoon heavy cream
- 1 tablespoon butter
- 1 teaspoon paprika
- ½ teaspoon nutmeg
- 1 teaspoon salt
- 1 teaspoon ground black pepper

Directions:

1. Chop the bacon into small pieces and sprinkle it with salt.
2. Mix to combine and put in the air fryer basket.
3. Preheat the air fryer to 360 F and cook the bacon for 5 minutes.
4. Meanwhile, crack the eggs in a bowl and whisk them using a hand whisker.
5. Sprinkle the egg mixture with paprika, nutmeg, and ground black pepper.
6. Whisk egg mixture gently.
7. Toss the butter into the bacon and pour the egg mixture.
8. Add the heavy cream and cook for 2 minutes.
9. Stir the mixture with a spatula until you get scrambled eggs and cook for 3 minutes more.
10. Transfer onto serving plates.

Nutrition: calories 387, fat 32.1,
fiber 0.4, carbs 2.3, protein 21.9

Cheddar Bacon Hash

Preparation time: 8 minutes
Cooking time: 8 minutes
Servings: 4
Ingredients:

- 1 zucchini
- 7 oz. bacon, cooked
- 4 oz. Cheddar cheese
- 2 tablespoon butter
- 1 teaspoon salt
- 1 teaspoon ground black pepper
- 1 teaspoon paprika
- 1 teaspoon cilantro
- 1 teaspoon ground thyme

Directions:

1. Chop the zucchini into the small cubes and sprinkle it with salt, ground black pepper, paprika, cilantro, and ground thyme.
2. Preheat the air fryer to 400 F and toss the butter into the air fryer basket tray.
3. Melt it and add the zucchini cubes.
4. Cook the zucchini for 5 minutes.
5. Meanwhile, shred Cheddar cheese.
6. Shake the zucchini cubes carefully and add the cooked bacon.
7. Sprinkle the zucchini mixture with the shredded cheese and cook it for 3 minutes more.
8. Transfer the breakfast hash in the serving bowls and stir.

Nutrition:
calories 445,
fat 36.1,
fiber 1,
carbs 3.5,
protein 26.3

Dinner

Thyme Turkey Breast

Preparation Time: 10 minutes
Cooking Time: 40 minutes
Serving: 4
Ingredients:

- 2 lb. turkey breast
- Salt, to taste
- Black pepper, to taste
- 4 tablespoon butter, melted
- 3 cloves garlic, minced
- 1 teaspoon thyme, chopped
- 1 teaspoon rosemary, chopped

Directions:

1. Mix butter with salt, black pepper, garlic, thyme, and rosemary in a bowl.
2. Rub this seasoning over the turkey breast liberally and place in the Air Fryer basket.
3. Turn the dial to select the "Air Fry" mode.
4. Hit the Time button and again use the dial to set the cooking time to 40 minutes
5. Now push the Temp button and rotate the dial to set the temperature at 375 degrees F.
6. Once preheated, place the Air fryer basket inside the oven

7. Slice and serve fresh.

Nutrition:
Calories 334
Fat 4.7 g
Carbs 54.1 g
Protein 26.2 g

Chicken Drumsticks

Basic Recipe
Preparation Time: 10 minutes
Cooking Time: 20 minutes
Serving: 8
Ingredients:

- 8 chicken drumsticks
- 2 tablespoon olive oil
- 1 teaspoon salt
- 1 teaspoon pepper
- 1 teaspoon garlic powder
- 1 teaspoon paprika
- 1/2 teaspoon cumin

Directions:

1. Mix olive oil with salt, black pepper, garlic powder, paprika, and cumin in a bowl.
2. Rub this mixture liberally over all the drumsticks.
3. Place these drumsticks in the Air fryer basket.
4. Turn the dial to select the "Air Fry" mode.
5. Hit the Time button and again use the dial to set the cooking time to 20 minutes
6. Now push the Temp button and rotate the dial to set the temperature at 375 degrees F.
7. Once preheated, place the Air fryer basket inside the oven.
8. Flip the drumsticks when cooked halfway through.

9. Resume air frying for another rest of the 10 minutes
10. Serve warm.

Nutrition:
Calories 212
Fat 11.8 g
Carbs 14.6 g
Protein 17.3 g

Blackened Chicken Bake

Basic Recipe
Preparation Time: 10 minutes
Cooking Time: 18 minutes
Serving: 4
Ingredients:

- 4 chicken breasts
- 2 teaspoon olive oil
- Seasoning:
- 1 1/2 tablespoon brown sugar
- 1 teaspoon paprika
- 1 teaspoon dried oregano
- 1/4 teaspoon garlic powder
- 1/2 teaspoon salt and pepper
- Garnish:
- Chopped parsley

Directions:

1. Mix olive oil with brown sugar, paprika, oregano, garlic powder, salt, and black pepper in a bowl.
2. Place the chicken breasts in the baking tray of the Ninja Oven.
3. Pour and rub this mixture liberally over all the chicken breasts.
4. Turn the dial to select the "Bake" mode.
5. Hit the Time button and again use the dial to set the cooking time to 18 minutes
6. Now push the Temp button and rotate the dial to set the temperature at 425 degrees F.

7. Once preheated, place the baking tray inside the oven
8. Serve warm.

Nutrition:
Calories 412
Fat 24.8 g
Carbs 43.8 g
Protein 18.9 g

Crusted Chicken Drumsticks
Basic Recipe
Preparation Time: 10 minutes
Cooking Time: 10 minutes
Serving: 4
Ingredients:

- 1 lb. chicken drumsticks
- 1/2 cup buttermilk
- 1/2 cup panko breadcrumbs
- 1/2 cup almond flour
- 1/4 teaspoon baking powder

Spice Mixture:

- 1/2 teaspoon salt
- 1/2 teaspoon celery salt
- 1/4 teaspoon oregano
- 1/4 teaspoon cayenne
- 1 teaspoon paprika
- 1/4 teaspoon garlic powder
- 1/4 teaspoon dried thyme
- 1/2 teaspoon ground ginger
- 1/2 teaspoon white pepper
- 1/2 teaspoon black pepper
- 3 tablespoon butter melted

Directions:

1. Soak chicken in the buttermilk and cover to marinate overnight in the refrigerator. Mix spices with flour, breadcrumbs, and baking powder in a shallow tray.
2. Remove the chicken from the milk and coat them well with the flour spice mixture
3. Place the chicken drumsticks in the Air fryer basket of the Ninja Oven.
4. Pour the melted butter over the drumsticks
5. Turn the dial to select the "Air fry" mode. Hit the Time button and again use the dial to set the cooking time to 10 minutes
6. Now push the Temp button and rotate the dial to set the temperature at 425 degrees F.
7. Once preheated, place the baking tray inside the oven
8. Flip the drumsticks and resume cooking for another 10 minutes
9. Serve warm.

Nutrition:
Calories 331
Fat 2.5 g
Carbs 69 g
Protein 28.7g

Brine Soaked Turkey
Intermediate Recipe
Preparation Time: 10 minutes
Cooking Time: 45 minutes
Serving: 8
Ingredients:

- 7 lb. bone-in, skin-on turkey breast
- Brine:
- 1/2 cup salt
- 1 lemon
- 1/2 onion
- 3 cloves garlic, smashed
- 5 sprigs fresh thyme
- 3 bay leaves

- Black pepper
- Turkey Breast:
- 4 tablespoon butter, softened
- 1/2 teaspoon black pepper
- 1/2 teaspoon garlic powder
- 1/4 teaspoon dried thyme
- 1/4 teaspoon dried oregano

Directions:

1. Mix the turkey brine ingredients in a pot and soak the turkey in the brine overnight. Next day, remove the soaked turkey from the brine.
2. Whisk the butter, black pepper, garlic powder, oregano, and thyme. Brush the butter mixture over the turkey then place it in a baking tray.
3. Press "Power Button" of Air Fry Oven and turn the dial to select the "Air Roast" mode. Press the Time button and again turn the dial to set the cooking time to 45 minutes
4. Now push the Temp button and rotate the dial to set the temperature at 370 degrees F. Once preheated, place the turkey baking tray in the oven and close its lid.
5. Slice and serve warm.

Nutrition:
Calories 397 Fat 15.4 g
Carbs 58.5 g Protein 7.9 g

Turkey Meatballs
Basic Recipe
Preparation Time: 10 minutes
Cooking Time: 20 minutes
Serving: 6
Ingredients:

- lb. turkey mince

- 1 red bell pepper, deseeded and chopped
- 1 large egg, beaten
- 4 tablespoons parsley, minced
- 1 tablespoon cilantro, minced
- Salt, to taste
- Black pepper, to taste

Directions:

1. Toss all the meatball ingredients in a bowl and mix well. Make small meatballs out this mixture and place them in the air fryer basket.
2. Press "Power Button" of Air Fry Oven and turn the dial to select the "Air Fry" mode. Press the Time button and again turn the dial to set the cooking time to 20 minutes
3. Now push the Temp button and rotate the dial to set the temperature at 375 degrees F.Once preheated, place the air fryer basket inside and close its lid. Serve warm.

Nutrition:
Calories 338
Fat 9.7 g
Carbs 32.5 g
Protein 10.3 g

Meat

Pecan Dijon Pork Chops
Preparation Time: 10 minutes
Cooking Time: 12 minutes
Servings: 6
Ingredients:

- 1 egg
- 6 pork chops, boneless

- 2 garlic cloves, minced
- 1 tablespoon water
- 1 teaspoon Dijon mustard
- 1 teaspoon garlic powder
- 1 teaspoon onion powder
- 2 teaspoon Italian seasoning
- 1/3 cup arrowroot
- 1 cup pecans, finely chopped
- 1/4 teaspoon salt

Directions:

1. In a shallow bowl, whisk the egg with garlic, water, and Dijon mustard.
2. In a separate shallow bowl, mix together arrowroot, pecans, Italian seasoning, onion powder, garlic powder, and salt.
3. Dip pork chop in the egg mixture and coat with arrowroot mixture.
4. Place the cooking tray in the air fryer basket.
5. Select Air Fry mode.
6. Set time to 12 minutes and temperature 400 F then press START.
7. The air fryer display will prompt you to ADD FOOD once the temperature is reached then place coated pork chops in the air fryer basket.
8. Turn pork chops halfway through.
9. Serve and enjoy.

Nutrition:

Calories 410

Fat 34.1 g

Carbohydrates 4.8 g

Sugar 1.1 g

Protein 21.4 g

Cholesterol 97 mg

Simple & Juicy Steak

Preparation Time: 10 minutes

Cooking Time: 13 minutes

Servings: 2

Ingredients:

- 12 oz ribeye steak
- 1 teaspoon steak seasoning
- 1 tablespoon olive oil
- Pepper
- Salt

Directions:

1. Coat steak with oil and season with steak seasoning, pepper, and salt.
2. Place the cooking tray in the air fryer basket.
3. Select Air Fry mode.
4. Set time to 13 minutes and temperature 400 F then press START.
5. The air fryer display will prompt you to ADD FOOD once the temperature is reached then place steak in the air fryer basket.
6. Serve and enjoy.

Nutrition:

Calories 241

Fat 11.6 g

Carbohydrates 0 g

Sugar 0 g

Protein 39.1 g

Cholesterol 90 mg

Marinated Ribeye Steaks

Preparation Time: 10 minutes

Cooking Time: 12 minutes

Servings: 4

Ingredients:

- 2 large ribeye steaks, 1 1/2-inch thick

- 1 1/2 tablespoon Montreal steak seasoning
- 1/2 cup low-sodium soy sauce
- 1/4 cup olive oil

Directions:

1. Add soy sauce, oil, and Montreal steak seasoning in a large zip-lock bag.
2. Add steaks in a zip-lock bag. Seal bag shakes well and places in the refrigerator for 2 hours.
3. Place the cooking tray in the air fryer basket.
4. Select Air Fry mode.
5. Set time to 12 minutes and temperature 400 F then press START.
6. The air fryer display will prompt you to ADD FOOD once the temperature is reached then remove steaks from marinade and place in the air fryer basket.
7. Turn steaks halfway through.
8. Serve and enjoy.

Nutrition:
Calories 186
Fat 14.1 g
Carbohydrates 2 g
Sugar 2 g
Protein 15 g
Cholesterol 30 mg

Fish

Moist & Juicy Baked Cod
Preparation Time: 10 minutes
Cooking Time: 10 minutes
Servings: 2
Ingredients:

- 1 lb cod fillets

- 1 1/2 tablespoon olive oil
- 3 dashes cayenne pepper
- 1 tablespoon lemon juice
- 1/4 teaspoon salt

Directions:

1. In a small bowl, mix together olive oil, cayenne pepper, lemon juice, and salt.
2. Brush fish fillets with oil mixture.
3. Place the cooking tray in the air fryer basket. Line air fryer basket with parchment paper.
4. Select Bake mode.
5. Set time to 10 minutes and temperature 400 F then press START.
6. The air fryer display will prompt you to ADD FOOD once the temperature is reached then place fish fillets in the air fryer basket.
7. Serve and enjoy.

Nutrition:
Calories 275
Fat 12.7 g
Carbohydrates 0.4 g
Sugar 0.2 g
Protein 40.6 g
Cholesterol 111 mg

Crunchy Fish Sticks
Preparation Time: 10 minutes
Cooking Time: 15 minutes
Servings: 5
Ingredients:

- 12 oz tilapia loins, cut into fish sticks

- 1/2 cup parmesan cheese, grated
- 3.25 oz pork rind, crushed
- 1 teaspoon paprika
- 1 teaspoon garlic powder
- 1/4 cup mayonnaise

Directions:

1. In a shallow bowl, mix together parmesan cheese, crushed pork rind, paprika, and garlic powder.
2. Add fish pieces and mayonnaise into the mixing bowl and mix well.
3. Place the cooking tray in the air fryer basket.
4. Select Air Fry mode.
5. Set time to 15 minutes and temperature 380 F then press START.
6. The air fryer display will prompt you to ADD FOOD once the temperature is reached then coat fish pieces with parmesan mixture and place in the air fryer basket.
7. Serve and enjoy.

Nutrition:
Calories 295
Fat 16.8 g
Carbohydrates 4.3 g
Sugar 0.9 g
Protein 33.4 g
Cholesterol 61 mg

Garlic Butter Fish Fillets

Preparation Time: 10 minutes
Cooking Time: 10 minutes
Servings: 2
Ingredients:

- 2 salmon fillets
- 1/4 teaspoon dried parsley
- 1 teaspoon garlic, minced
- 2 tablespoon butter, melted
- Pepper
- Salt

Directions:

1. In a small bowl, mix together melted butter, garlic, and parsley.
2. Season fish fillets with pepper and salt and brush with melted butter mixture.
3. Place the cooking tray in the air fryer basket.
4. Select Air Fry mode.
5. Set time to 10 minutes and temperature 360 F then press START.
6. The air fryer display will prompt you to ADD FOOD once the temperature is reached then place fish fillets skin side down in the air fryer basket.
7. Serve and enjoy.

Nutrition:
Calories 340
Fat 22.5 g
Carbohydrates 0.5 g
Sugar 0 g
Protein 34.8 g
Cholesterol 109 mg

<u>Vegetable</u>

Crisp & Crunchy Asparagus
Preparation Time: 10 minutes
Cooking Time: 10 minutes
Servings: 4
Ingredients:

- 1 lb asparagus, trim ends & cut in half
- 1 tablespoon vinegar
- 2 tablespoon coconut aminos
- 1 tablespoon butter, melted
- 1 tablespoon olive oil
- 1/2 teaspoon sea salt

Directions:

1. In a bowl, toss asparagus with olive oil and salt.
2. Place the cooking tray in the air fryer basket.
3. Select Air Fry mode.
4. Set time to 10 minutes and temperature 400 F then press START.
5. The air fryer display will prompt you to ADD FOOD once the temperature is reached then add asparagus in the air fryer basket.
6. Meanwhile, for the sauce in a bowl, mix together coconut aminos, melted butter, and vinegar.
7. Pour sauce over hot asparagus and serve.

Nutrition:
Calories 86
Fat 6.5 g
Carbohydrates 5.9 g
Sugar 2.2 g
Protein 2.5 g
Cholesterol 8 mg

Balsamic Brussels Sprouts
Preparation Time: 10 minutes
Cooking Time: 20 minutes
Servings: 4
Ingredients:

- 1 lb brussels sprouts, cut in half
- 1 small onion, sliced
- 3 bacon slices, cut into pieces
- 1 teaspoon garlic powder
- 2 tablespoon fresh lemon juice
- 2 tablespoon balsamic vinegar
- 3 tablespoon olive oil
- 1/2 teaspoon sea salt

Directions:

1. In a small bowl, whisk together balsamic vinegar, olive oil, lemon juice, garlic powder, and salt.
2. Toss brussels sprouts with 3 tablespoons of the balsamic vinegar mixture.
3. Place the cooking tray in the air fryer basket.
4. Select Air Fry mode.
5. Set time to 20 minutes and temperature 370 F then press START.
6. The air fryer display will prompt you to ADD FOOD once the temperature is reached then add brussels sprouts in the air fryer basket.
7. After 10 minutes toss Brussels sprouts and top with bacon and onion and air fry for 10 minutes more.

8. Drizzle remaining balsamic vinegar mixture over brussels sprouts and serve.

Nutrition:
Calories 229
Fat 16.9 g
Carbohydrates 12.9 g
Sugar 3.6 g
Protein 9.5 g
Cholesterol 16 mg

Roasted Radishes

Preparation Time: 10 minutes

Cooking Time: 30 minutes

Serve: 2

Ingredients:

- 3 cups radish, clean and halved
- 8 black peppercorns, crushed
- 3 tbsp olive oil
- 2 tbsp fresh rosemary, chopped
- 2 tsp sea salt

Directions:

1. Add radishes, salt, peppercorns, rosemary, and 2 tablespoons of olive oil in a bowl and toss well.
2. Pour radishes mixture onto the cooking tray.
3. Select BAKE mode, then set the temperature to 400 F and the time to 30 minutes, then press start.
4. When the display shows Add Food then place the cooking tray in the vortex plus air fryer oven.
5. Heat remaining olive oil in a pan over medium heat.
6. Add baked radishes in the pan and sauté for 2 minutes.
7. Serve and enjoy.

Nutrition:
Calories 220
Fat 21.7 g
Carbohydrates 8.3 g
Sugar 3.2 g
Protein 1.4 g
Cholesterol 0 mg

Parmesan Zucchini Noodles

Preparation Time: 10 minutes
Cooking Time: 10 minutes
Servings: 2
Ingredients:

- 4 cups zucchini noodles
- 1/2 cup parmesan cheese, grated
- 2 tablespoon mayonnaise

Directions:

1. Add zucchini noodles into the microwave-safe bowl and microwave for 3 minutes. Pat dry zucchini noodles with a paper towel.
2. In a mixing bowl, toss zucchini noodles with parmesan cheese and mayonnaise.
3. Place the cooking tray in the air fryer basket. Line air fryer basket with parchment paper.
4. Select Air Fry mode.
5. Set time to 10 minutes and temperature 400 F then press START.

6. The air fryer display will prompt you to ADD FOOD once the temperature is reached then add zucchini noodles onto the parchment paper in the air fryer basket. Stir zucchini noodles halfway through.
7. Serve and enjoy.

Nutrition:
Calories 261
Fat 17.6 g
Carbohydrates 8.9 g
Sugar 2.6 g
Protein 20.1 g
Cholesterol 46 mg

Snacks

Parsley Shrimp Tails
Preparation time: 10 minutes
Cooking time: 14 minutes
Servings: 6
Ingredients:
- 1-pound shrimp tails
- 1 tablespoon olive oil
- 1 teaspoon dried dill
- ½ teaspoon dried parsley
- 2 tablespoon coconut flour
- ½ cup heavy cream
- 1 teaspoon chili flakes

Directions:
1. Peel the shrimp tails and sprinkle them with the dried dill and dried parsley.
2. Mix the shrimp tails carefully in a mixing bowl.
3. Combine the coconut flour, heavy cream, and chili flakes in a separate bowl and whisk until smooth.
4. Preheat the air fryer to 330 F.
5. Place the shrimp tails in the cream mix and stir.
6. Grease the air fryer rack and put the shrimp tails inside.
7. Cook the shrimp tails for 7 minutes.
8. Turn the shrimp.
9. Cook the shrimp tails for 7 minutes more.

Nutrition:
calories 155,
fat 7.6,
fiber 1,
carbs 3.2,
protein 17.8

Calamari Almond Rings
Preparation time: 12 minutes
Cooking time: 8 minutes
Servings: 4
Ingredients:
- 1 cup almond flour
- 9 oz. calamari
- 1 egg
- ½ teaspoon lemon zest
- 1 teaspoon fresh lemon juice
- ½ teaspoon turmeric
- ¼ teaspoon salt

- ¼ teaspoon ground black pepper

Directions:

1. Wash and peel the calamari.
2. Slice the calamari into thick rings.
3. Crack the egg in a bowl and whisk it.
4. Add lemon zest, turmeric, salt, and ground black pepper to the bowl and mix.
5. Sprinkle the calamari rings with fresh lemon juice.
6. Place the calamari rings in the whisked egg and stir.
7. Leave the calamari rings in the egg mixture for 4 minutes.
8. Coat the calamari rings in the almond flour mixture well.
9. Preheat the air fryer to 360 F.
10. Transfer the calamari rings to the air fryer rack.
11. Cook the calamari rings for 8 minutes.

Nutrition:
calories 190,
fat 15.7,
fiber 3.1,
carbs 7,
protein 8.7

Keto Beef Bombs
Preparation time: 15 minutes

Cooking time: 14 minutes
Servings: 7
Ingredients:

- 6 oz. ground chicken
- 6 oz. ground beef
- 6 oz. ground pork
- 2 oz chive stems
- 3 garlic cloves, minced
- 1 tablespoon dried parsley
- ½ teaspoon salt
- ½ teaspoon chili flakes
- 1 egg
- 1 tablespoon butter

Directions:

1. Put the ground chicken, ground beef, and ground pork in a mixing bowl.
2. Add the diced chives, minced garlic, dried parsley, salt, and chili flakes.
3. Crack the egg into the bowl with the ground meat.
4. Stir the meat mixture using your hands.
5. Melt butter and add it to the ground meat mixture.
6. Stir.
7. Leave the ground meat mixture for 5 minutes to rest.
8. Preheat the air fryer to 370 F.
9. Make small meatballs from the meat mixture and put them in the air fryer.
10. Cook the meatballs for 14 minutes.

11. Cool before serving.

Nutrition:
calories 155,
fat 6.5,
fiber 0.2,
carbs 1.3,
protein 21.8

Paprika Mozzarella Balls

Preparation time: 10 minutes
Cooking time: 10 minutes
Servings: 6
Ingredients:

- 5 oz. bacon, sliced
- 10 oz. mozzarella
- ¼ teaspoon ground black pepper
- ¼ teaspoon paprika

Directions:

1. Sprinkle the sliced bacon with ground black pepper and paprika.
2. Wrap the mozzarella balls in the bacon.
3. Secure the mozzarella balls with toothpicks.
4. Preheat the air fryer to 360 F.
5. Put the mozzarella balls in the air fryer rack and cook for 10 minutes.

Nutrition:
calories 262, fat 18.2,
fiber 0.1, carbs 2.1,
protein 22.1

Dessert

Coconut Muffins

Preparation Time: 5 minutes
Cooking time: 25 minutes
Servings: 5
Ingredients:

- ½ cup coconut flour
- 2 tablespoons cocoa powder
- 3 tablespoons Erythritol
- 1 teaspoon baking powder
- 2 tablespoons coconut oil
- 2 eggs, beaten
- ½ cup coconut shred

Directions:

1. In the mixing bowl, mix all ingredients.
2. Then pour the mixture in the molds of the muffin and transfer in the air fryer basket.
3. Cook the muffins at 350F for 25 minutes.

Nutrition:
calories 206, fat 16.7,
fiber 7.1, carbs 13,
protein 4.2

Coffee Muffins

Preparation time: 10 minutes
Cooking time: 11 minutes
Servings: 6
Ingredients:

- 1 cup coconut flour
- 4 tablespoons coconut oil
- 1 teaspoon vanilla extract
- 1 teaspoon instant coffee
- 1 teaspoon baking powder
- 1 egg, beaten
- ¼ cup Erythritol

Directions:

1. Mix coconut flour with coconut oil, vanilla extract, instant coffee, baking powder, egg, and Erythritol.
2. Put the mixture in the muffin molds and cook in the air fryer at 375F for 11 minutes.

Nutrition:
calories 172,
fat 11.8,
fiber 8,
carbs 13.9,
protein 3.6

Almond Cookies

Preparation Time: 5 minutes
Cooking time: 15 minutes
Servings: 8
Ingredients:

- 1 cup almond flour
- 2 oz almonds, grinded
- 2 tablespoons Erythritol
- ½ teaspoon baking powder
- 5 tablespoons coconut oil, softened
- ½ teaspoon vanilla extract

Directions:

1. Mix almond flour with almonds, Erythritol, baking powder, coconut oil, and vanilla extract. Knead the dough.
2. Make the small cookies and place them in the air fryer basket.
3. Cook the cookies at 350F for 15 minutes.

Nutrition:
calories 199, fat 18.7,
fiber 2.4, carbs 4.7,
 protein 4.5

Thumbprint Cookies

Preparation time: 15 minutes
Cooking time: 9 minutes
Servings: 6
Ingredients:

- 2 teaspoons coconut oil, softened
- 1 tablespoon Erythritol
- 1 egg, beaten
- ½ cup coconut flour
- 1 oz almonds, chopped

Directions:

1. Mix all ingredients in the mixing bowl. Knead the dough.
2. Then make cookies from the dough and put in the air fryer basket.
3. Cook the cookies at 365F for 9 minutes.

Nutrition:
calories 91,
fat 5.6,
fiber 4.6,
carbs 10.2,
protein 3.3

Pecan Bars

Preparation Time: 5 minutes
Cooking time: 40 minutes
Servings: 12
Ingredients:

- 2 cups coconut flour
- 5 tablespoons Erythritol
- 4 tablespoons coconut oil, softened
- ½ cup heavy cream
- 1 egg, beaten
- 4 pecans, chopped

Directions:

1. Mix coconut flour, Erythritol, coconut oil, heavy cream, and egg.
2. Pour the batter in the air fryer basket and flatten well.
3. Top the mixture with pecans and cook the meal at 350F for 40 minutes.
4. Cut the cooked meal into the bars.

Nutrition:
calories 174,
fat 12.1,
fiber 8.5,
carbs 14.2,
protein 3.7

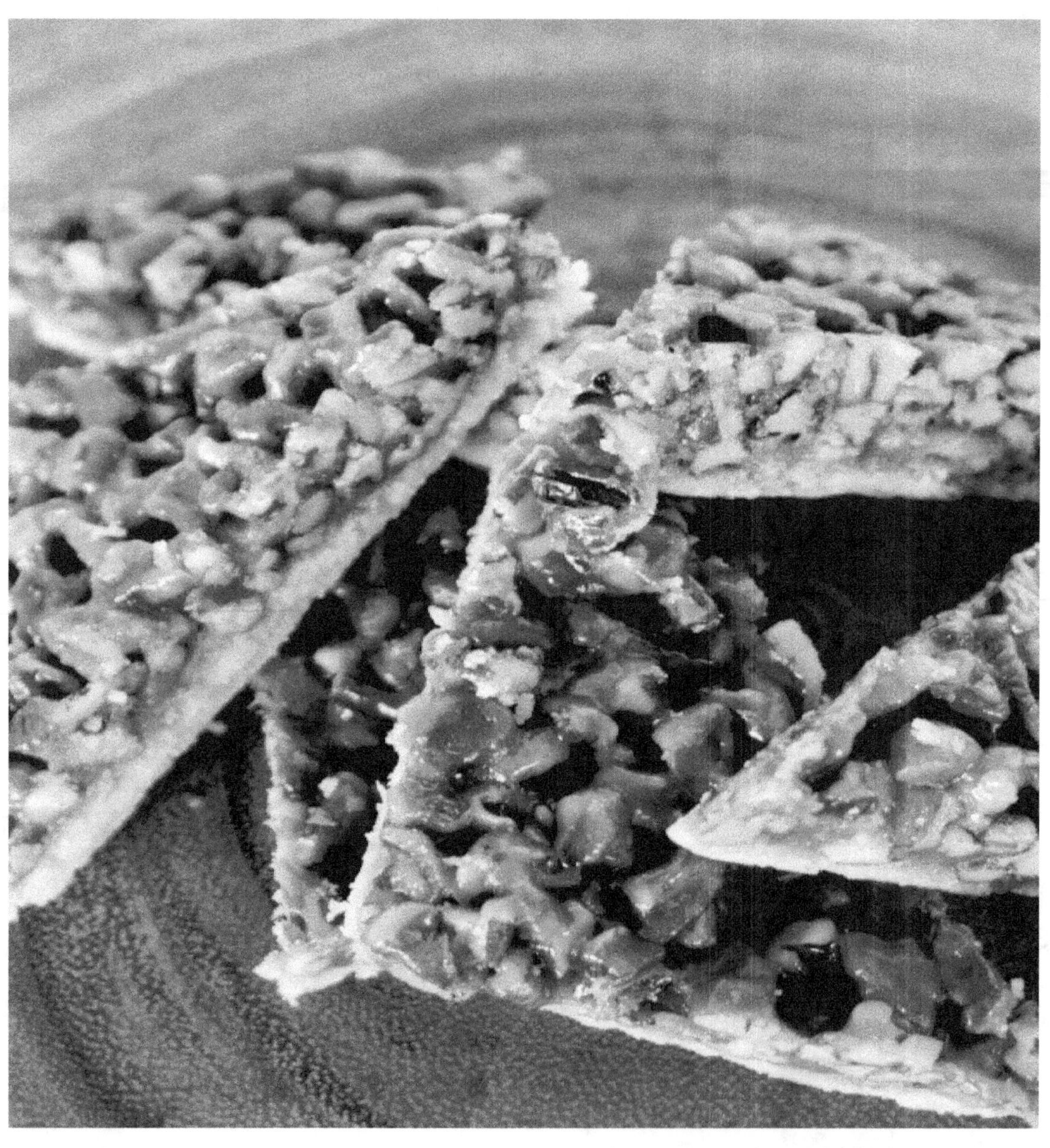

CHAPTER 4:

February

Lunch

Egg Clouds
Preparation time: 8 minutes
Cooking time: 4 minutes
Servings: 2
Ingredients:
- 2 eggs
- 1 teaspoon butter

Directions:
1. Separate the egg whites and egg yolks into separate bowls.
2. Whisk the egg whites with a hand mixer until you get strong white peaks.
3. Grease the Air Fryer basket tray with butter.
4. Preheat the Air Fryer to 300 F.
5. Make the medium clouds from the egg white peaks in the Prepared Air Fryer basket tray.
6. Place the basket tray in the Air Fryer and cook the cloud eggs for 2 minutes.
7. Remove the basket from the Air Fryer, place the egg yolks in the center of every egg cloud, and return the basket back in the Air Fryer.
8. Cook the dish for 2 minutes.
9. Remove the cooked dish from the basket and serve.

Nutrition:
calories 80,
fat 6.3,
fiber 0,
carbs 0.3,
protein 5.6

Flax & Chia Porridge
Preparation time: 5 minutes
Cooking time: 8 minutes
Servings: 7
Ingredients:
- 2 tablespoon sesame seeds
- 4 tablespoon chia seeds
- 1 cup almond milk
- 3 tablespoon flax meal
- 1 teaspoon stevia
- 1 tablespoon butter
- ½ teaspoon vanilla extract

Directions:
1. Preheat the air fryer to 375 F.
2. Put the sesame seeds, chia seeds, almond milk, flax meal, stevia, and butter in the air fryer basket tray.
3. Add the vanilla extract and cook the porridge for 8 minutes.
4. Stir the porridge carefully and leave it for 5 minutes to rest.

5. Transfer to serving bowls or ramekins.

Nutrition:
calories 198,
fat 21.7,
fiber 6.4,
carbs 8.3,
protein 4.8

Parmesan Ham Hash

Preparation time: 10 minutes
Cooking time: 10 minutes
Servings: 6
Ingredients:

- 5 oz. Parmesan
- 10 oz. ham
- 1 tablespoon butter
- 3 oz chive stems
- 1 teaspoon ground black pepper
- 1 egg
- 1 teaspoon paprika

Directions:

1. Grate Parmesan cheese.
2. Cut the ham into small strips.
3. Dice the chive stems.
4. Crack the egg in a bowl and whisk with a hand whisker.
5. Add the ham strips, butter, diced chives, and butter.
6. Sprinkle the mixture with the ground black pepper and paprika.
7. Mix well.
8. Preheat Air Fryer to 350 F.
9. Transfer the ham mixture into 3 ramekins and sprinkle them with the grated Parmesan cheese.
10. Place the ramekins in the preheated Air Fryer and cook them for 10 minutes.
11. Remove the ramekins from the Air Fryer and mix the ham hash with a fork.
12. Serve the dish.

Nutrition:
calories 186,
fat 12,
fiber 1,
carbs 4,
protein 16.7

Paprika Eggs with Bacon

Preparation time: 10 minutes
Cooking time: 15 minutes
Servings: 4
Ingredients:

- 4 eggs
- 6 oz. bacon
- ¼ teaspoon salt
- ½ teaspoon dried dill
- ½ teaspoon paprika
- 1 tablespoon butter

Directions:

1. Crack the eggs in a mixer bowl.
2. Add salt, dried dill, and paprika. Mix the egg mixture carefully with a hand mixer.
3. Grease 4 ramekins with butter.

4. Slice the bacon and put it in the Preparationared ramekins in the shape of cups.

5. Pour the egg mixture in the middle of each bacon cup.

6. Set the Air Fryer to 360 F.

7. Put the ramekins in the Air Fryer and close it.

8. Cook the dish for 15 minutes.

9. Remove the egg cups from the Air Fryer and serve them.

Nutrition:
calories 319,
fat 25.1,
fiber 0.1,
carbs 1.2,
protein 21.4

Eggs in Avocado

Preparation time: 8 minutes
Cooking time: 15 minutes
Servings: 2
Ingredients:

- 1 avocado, pitted
- ¼ teaspoon turmeric
- ¼ teaspoon ground black pepper
- ¼ teaspoon salt
- 2 eggs
- 1 teaspoon butter
- ¼ teaspoon flax seeds

Directions:

1. Take a shallow bowl and add the turmeric, ground black pepper, salt, and flax seeds together. Shake gently to combine.

2. Cut the avocado into 2 halves.

3. Crack the eggs in a separate bowl.

4. Sprinkle the eggs with the spice mixture.

5. Place the eggs in the avocado halves.

6. Put the avocado boats in the Air Fryer.

7. Set the Air Fryer to 355 F and close it.

8. Cook the dish for 15 minutes or until the eggs are cooked to preference.

9. Serve immediately.

Nutrition:
calories 288,
fat 26,
fiber 6.9,
carbs 9.4,
protein 7.6

Baked Cheddar Egg Cups

Preparation time: 10 minutes
Cooking time: 12 minutes
Servings: 2
Ingredients:

- 2 eggs
- 4 oz. bacon
- ¼ teaspoon salt
- ½ teaspoon butter
- 3 oz. Cheddar cheese, shredded
- ½ teaspoon cayenne pepper
- ½ teaspoon paprika
- 1 tablespoon chives

Directions:

1. Chop the bacon into small pieces and sprinkle it with salt, cayenne pepper, and paprika.
2. Mix well to combine.
3. Grease the ramekins with butter and crack the eggs dividing between the cups.
4. Add the shredded cheese and chives.
5. Add the chopped bacon over the chives.
6. Put the ramekins in the Air Fryer basket and preheat the air fryer to 360 F.
7. Put the air fryer basket in the air fryer and cook for 12 minutes.
8. Remove the ramekins from the air fryer to chill.
9. Remove the bacon egg cups from the ramekins carefully.

Nutrition:
calories 553, fat 43.3,
fiber 0.4, carbs 2.3, protein 37.3

Cauliflower Fritters

Preparation time: 10 minutes
Cooking time: 15 minutes
Servings: 4
Ingredients:

- 1 tablespoon dried dill
- 1 egg
- 1 teaspoon salt
- 10 oz. cauliflower
- 1 tablespoon almond flour
- 1 teaspoon olive oil
- 1 tablespoon parsley
- ½ teaspoon ground white pepper

Directions:

1. Wash the cauliflower carefully and chop it into small pieces.
2. Place the cauliflower in a blender and blend well.
3. Crack the egg in the cauliflower mixture and continue to blend for 1 minute.
4. Transfer the blended cauliflower mixture into a bowl.
5. Sprinkle with the salt, dried dill, almond flour, parsley, and ground white pepper.
6. Mix carefully using a spoon.
7. Preheat the air fryer to 355 F.
8. Grease the air fryer basket tray with olive oil.
9. Form the cauliflower mixture into four patties using your hands and put them in the air fryer basket tray.
10. Close the air fryer and cook the fritters for 8 minutes.
11. Turn the fritters over and cook them for a further 7 minutes.
12. Serve hot.

Nutrition:
calories 54, fat 3.1, fiber 2.1,
carbs 4.8,
protein 3.3

Dinner

Ground Chicken Meatballs
Basic Recipe
Preparation Time: 10 minutes
Cooking Time: 10 minutes
Serving: 4
Ingredients:

- 1-lb. ground chicken
- 1/3 cup panko
- 1 teaspoon salt
- 2 teaspoons chives
- 1/2 teaspoon garlic powder
- 1 teaspoon thyme
- 1 egg

Directions:

1. Toss all the meatball ingredients in a bowl and mix well. Make small meatballs out this mixture and place them in the air fryer basket.
2. Press "Power Button" of Air Fry Oven and turn the dial to select the "Air Fry" mode.Press the Time button and again turn the dial to set the cooking time to 10 minutes
3. Now push the Temp button and rotate the dial to set the temperature at 350 degrees F.Once preheated, place the air fryer basket inside and close its lid. Serve warm.

Nutrition:
Calories 453
Fat 2.4 g
Carbs 18 g
Protein 23.2 g

Parmesan Chicken Meatballs
Basic Recipe
Preparation Time: 10 minutes
Cooking Time: 12 minutes
Serving: 4
Ingredients:

- 1-lb. ground chicken
- 1 large egg, beaten
- ½ cup Parmesan cheese, grated
- ½ cup pork rinds, ground
- 1 teaspoon garlic powder
- 1 teaspoon paprika
- 1 teaspoon kosher salt
- ½ teaspoon pepper

Crust:

- ½ cup pork rinds, ground

Directions:

1. Toss all the meatball ingredients in a bowl and mix well.Make small meatballs out this mixture and roll them in the pork rinds.
2. Place the coated meatballs in the air fryer basket.Press "Power Button" of Air Fry Oven and turn the dial to select the "Bake" mode.
3. Press the Time button and again turn the dial to set the cooking time to 12 minutes. Now push the Temp button and rotate the dial to set the temperature at 400 degrees F.
4. Once preheated, place the air fryer basket inside and close its lid.
5. Serve warm.

Nutrition:
Calories 529
Fat 17 g
Carbs 55 g
Protein 41g

Easy Italian Meatballs

Basic Recipe
Preparation Time: 10 minutes
Cooking Time: 13 minutes
Serving: 4
Ingredients:

- 2-lb. lean ground turkey
- ¼ cup onion, minced
- 2 cloves garlic, minced
- 2 tablespoons parsley, chopped
- 2 eggs
- 1½ cup parmesan cheese, grated
- ½ teaspoon red pepper flakes
- ½ teaspoon Italian seasoning
- Salt and black pepper to taste

Directions:

1. Toss all the meatball ingredients in a bowl and mix well. Make small meatballs out this mixture and place them in the air fryer basket.
2. Press "Power Button" of Air Fry Oven and turn the dial to select the "Air Fry" mode. Press the Time button and again turn the dial to set the cooking time to 13 minutes. Now push the Temp button and rotate the dial to set the temperature at 350 degrees F.
3. Once preheated, place the air fryer basket inside and close its lid.
4. Flip the meatballs when cooked halfway through.
5. Serve warm.

Nutrition:
Calories 472
Fat 25.8
Carbs 1.7 g
Protein 59.6 g

Oregano Chicken Breast

Basic Recipe
Preparation Time: 10 minutes
Cooking Time: 25 minutes
Serving: 6
Ingredients:

- 2 lbs. chicken breasts, minced
- 1 tablespoon avocado oil
- 1 teaspoon smoked paprika
- 1 teaspoon garlic powder
- 1 teaspoon oregano
- 1/2 teaspoon salt
- Black pepper, to taste

Directions:

1. Toss all the meatball ingredients in a bowl and mix well. Make small meatballs out this mixture and place them in the air fryer basket.
2. Press "Power Button" of Air Fry Oven and turn the dial to select the "Air Fry" mode. Press the Time button and again turn the dial to set the cooking time to 25 minutes
3. Now push the Temp button and rotate the dial to set the temperature at 375 degrees F.
4. Once preheated, place the air fryer basket inside and close its lid.
5. Serve warm.

Nutrition:
Calories 352
Fat 14 g
Carbs: 15.8 g
Protein 26 g

Lemon Chicken Breasts

Basic Recipe
Preparation Time: 10 minutes
Cooking Time: 30 minutes
Serving: 4
Ingredients:

- 1/4 cup olive oil
- 3 tablespoons garlic, minced
- 1/3 cup dry white wine
- 1 tablespoon lemon zest, grated
- 2 tablespoons lemon juice
- 1 1/2 teaspoons dried oregano, crushed
- 1 teaspoon thyme leaves, minced
- Salt and black pepper
- 4 skin-on boneless chicken breasts
- 1 lemon, sliced

Directions:

1. Whisk everything in a baking pan to coat the chicken breasts well.
2. Place the lemon slices on top of the chicken breasts.
3. Spread the mustard mixture over the toasted bread slices.
4. Press "Power Button" of Air Fry Oven and turn the dial to select the "Bake" mode.
5. Press the Time button and again turn the dial to set the cooking time to 30 minutes
6. Now push the Temp button and rotate the dial to set the temperature at 370 degrees F.
7. Once preheated, place the baking pan inside and close its lid.
8. Serve warm.

Nutrition:
Calories 388 Fat 8 g
Carbs 8 g Protein 13 g

Cajun Salmon

Basic Recipe
Preparation Time: 5 minutes
Cooking Time: 10 minutes
Serving: 2
Ingredients:

- 2 Salmon steaks
- 2 tbspcajun seasoning

Directions:

1. Rub the salmon steaks with the Cajun seasoning evenly. Set aside for about 10 minutes. Arrange the salmon steaks onto the greased cooking tray.
2. Arrange the drip pan in the bottom of the Instant Vortex Air Fryer Oven cooking chamber. Select "Air Fry" and then adjust the temperature to 390 °F. Set the time for 8 minutes and press "Start".
3. When the display shows "Add Food" insert the cooking tray in the center position. When the display shows "Turn Food" turn the salmon steaks.
4. When the cooking time is complete, remove the tray from the Vortex Oven. Serve hot.

Nutrition:
Calories 225
Carbs 0g
Fat 10.5g
Protein 22.1g

Meat

Pork Chop Fries

Preparation Time: 10 minutes
Cooking Time: 15 minutes
Servings: 4
Ingredients:

- 1 lb pork chops, cut into fries
- 1/2 cup parmesan cheese, grated
- 3.5 oz pork rinds, crushed
- 1/2 cup ranch dressing
- Pepper
- Salt

Directions

1. In a shallow dish, mix together crushed pork rinds, parmesan cheese, pepper, and salt.
2. Add pork chop pieces and ranch dressing into the zip-lock bag, seal bag, and shake well.
3. Remove pork chop pieces from zip-lock bag and coat with crushed pork rind mixture.
4. Place the cooking tray in the air fryer basket. Line air fryer basket with parchment paper.
5. Select Bake mode.
6. Set time to 15 minutes and temperature 400 F then press START.
7. The air fryer display will prompt you to ADD FOOD once the temperature is reached then place breaded pork chop fries in the air fryer basket.
8. Serve and enjoy.

Nutrition:
Calories 608 Fat 43.4 g
Carbohydrates 2.7 g Sugar 0.8 g
Protein 51.2 g Cholesterol 154 mg

Pork Kebabs

Preparation Time: 10 minutes
Cooking Time: 15 minutes
Servings: 6
Ingredients:

- 2 lbs country-style pork ribs, cut into cubes
- 1/4 cup soy sauce
- 1/2 cup olive oil
- 1 tablespoon Italian seasoning

Directions

1. Add soy sauce, oil, Italian seasoning, and pork cubes into the zip-lock bag, seal bag and place in the refrigerator for 4 hours.
2. Remove pork cubes from marinade and place the cubes on wooden skewers.
3. Place the cooking tray in the air fryer basket. Line air fryer basket with parchment paper.
4. Select Bake mode.
5. Set time to 15 minutes and temperature 380 F then press START.
6. The air fryer display will prompt you to ADD FOOD once the temperature is reached then place pork skewers in the air fryer basket.
7. Serve and enjoy.

Nutrition:
Calories 438
Fat 34.9 g
Carbohydrates 1.1 g
Sugar 0.4 g
Protein 30.1 g
Cholesterol 115 mg

Feta Cheese Meatballs

Preparation Time: 10 minutes
Cooking Time: 12 minutes
Servings: 8
Ingredients:

- 2 lbs ground pork
- 2 eggs, lightly beaten
- 1/4 cup fresh parsley, chopped
- 1 tablespoon garlic, minced
- 1 onion, chopped
- 1 tablespoon Worcestershire sauce
- 1/2 cup feta cheese, crumbled
- 1/2 cup almond flour
- Pepper
- Salt

Directions:

1. Add all ingredients into the mixing bowl and mix until well combined.
2. Make small balls from the meat mixture.
3. Select Air Fry mode.
4. Set time to 12 minutes and temperature 400 F then press START.
5. The air fryer display will prompt you to ADD FOOD once the temperature is reached then place meatballs in the air fryer basket.
6. Serve and enjoy.

Nutrition:
Calories 222
Fat 8 g
Carbohydrates 3 g
Sugar 1.5 g
Protein 33.1 g
Cholesterol 132 mg

Fish

Baked Tilapia

Preparation Time: 10 minutes
Cooking Time: 15 minutes
Servings: 6
Ingredients:

- 6 tilapia fillets
- 1/2 cup Asiago cheese, grated
- 1/4 teaspoon basil
- 1/4 teaspoon thyme
- 1/4 teaspoon onion powder
- 1 teaspoon garlic, minced
- 1/2 cup mayonnaise
- 1/8 teaspoon pepper
- 1/4 teaspoon salt

Directions:

1. In a small bowl, mix together the grated cheese, basil, thyme, onion powder, garlic, mayonnaise, pepper, and salt.
2. Place the cooking tray in the air fryer basket. Line air fryer basket with parchment paper.
3. Select Bake mode.
4. Set time to 15 minutes and temperature 350 F then press START.
5. The air fryer display will prompt you to ADD FOOD once the temperature is reached then place fish fillets in the air fryer basket and spread cheese mixture on top of each fish fillet.
6. Serve and enjoy.

Nutrition:
Calories 287 Fat 13.7 g
Carbohydrates 5 g Sugar 1.3 g
Protein 36.7 g Cholesterol 105 mg

Baked Parmesan Tilapia

Preparation Time: 10 minutes
Cooking Time: 10 minutes
Servings: 4
Ingredients:

- 2 lbs tilapia
- 1/4 teaspoon paprika
- 1/4 teaspoon dried basil
- 2 garlic cloves, minced
- 1 teaspoon dried parsley
- 1 tablespoon butter, softened
- 2 tablespoon fresh lemon juice
- 1/4 cup mayonnaise
- 1/2 cup parmesan cheese, grated
- 1/2 teaspoon salt

Directions:

1. In a small bowl, mix together parmesan cheese, mayonnaise, lemon juice, butter, parsley, garlic, basil, paprika, and salt.
2. Place the cooking tray in the air fryer basket. Line air fryer basket with parchment paper.
3. Select Bake mode.
4. Set time to 10 minutes and temperature 400 F then press START.
5. The air fryer display will prompt you to ADD FOOD once the temperature is reached then place fish fillets in the air fryer basket and spread the parmesan mixture on top of each fish fillet.
6. Serve and enjoy.

Nutrition:
Calories 368 Fat 16.2 g
Carbohydrates 5.3 g
Sugar 1.1 g Protein 51.9 g
Cholesterol 143 mg

Vegetable

Rosemary Basil Mushrooms

Preparation Time: 10 minutes
Cooking Time: 14 minutes
Servings: 4
Ingredients:

- 1 lb mushrooms
- 1/2 tablespoon vinegar
- 1/2 teaspoon ground coriander
- 1 teaspoon rosemary, chopped
- 1 tablespoon basil, minced
- 1 garlic clove, minced
- Pepper
- Salt

Directions:

1. Add all ingredients into the large bowl and toss well.
2. Select Air Fry mode.
3. Set time to 14 minutes and temperature 350 F then press START.
4. The air fryer display will prompt you to ADD FOOD once the temperature is reached then add mushrooms in the air fryer basket.
5. Serve and enjoy.

Nutrition:
Calories 27
Fat 0.4 g
Carbohydrates 4.2 g
Sugar 2 g
Protein 3.6 g
Cholesterol 0 mg

Baked Brussels Sprouts

Preparation Time: 10 minutes
Cooking Time: 35 minutes
Servings: 6
Ingredients:

- 2 cups Brussels sprouts, halved
- 1/4 teaspoon garlic powder
- 1/4 cup olive oil
- 1/2 teaspoon cayenne pepper
- 1/4 teaspoon salt

Directions:

1. Add all ingredients into the large bowl and toss well.
2. Select Bake mode.
3. Set time to 35 minutes and temperature 400 F then press START.
4. The air fryer display will prompt you to ADD FOOD once the temperature is reached then add brussels sprouts in the air fryer basket.
5. Serve and enjoy.

Nutrition:
Calories 86
Fat 8.5 g
Carbohydrates 2.8 g
Sugar 0.7 g
Protein 1 g
Cholesterol 0 mg

Old Bay Cauliflower Florets

Preparation Time: 10 minutes
Cooking Time: 15 minutes
Servings: 4
Ingredients:

- 1 medium cauliflower head, cut into florets
- 1/2 teaspoon old bay seasoning
- 1/4 teaspoon paprika
- 1 tablespoon garlic, minced
- 3 tablespoon olive oil
- Pepper
- Salt

Directions:

1. In a large bowl, toss cauliflower with remaining ingredients.
2. Select Air Fry mode.
3. Set time to 15 minutes and temperature 400 F then press START.
4. The air fryer display will prompt you to ADD FOOD once the temperature is reached then add cauliflower florets in the air fryer basket.
5. Serve and enjoy.

Nutrition:
Calories 130
Fat 10.7 g
Carbohydrates 8.4 g
Sugar 3.5 g
Protein 3 g
Cholesterol 0 mg

Rosemary Mushrooms

Preparation Time: 10 minutes
Cooking Time: 14 minutes
Servings: 4
Ingredients:

- 1 lb mushroom caps
- 1/2 teaspoon ground coriander
- 1 teaspoon rosemary, chopped
- 1/2 teaspoon garlic powder
- Pepper
- Salt

Directions:

1. Add all ingredients into the mixing bowl and toss well.
2. Select Air Fry mode.

3. Set time to 14 minutes and temperature 350 F then press START.
4. The air fryer display will prompt you to ADD FOOD once the temperature is reached then add mushrooms in the air fryer basket.
5. Serve and enjoy.

Nutrition:
Calories 27
Fat 0.4 g
Carbohydrates 4.2 g
Sugar 2 g
Protein 3.6 g
Cholesterol 0 mg

Snacks

Toasted Macadamia & Nuts Mix
Preparation time: 5 minutes
Cooking time: 9 minutes
Servings: 4
Ingredients:

- ¼ cup hazelnuts
- ¼ cup walnuts
- ½ cup pecans
- ½ cup macadamia nuts
- 1 tablespoon olive oil
- 1 teaspoon salt

Directions:
1. Preheat the air fryer to 320 F.
2. Place the hazelnuts, walnuts, pecans, and macadamia nuts in the air fryer.
3. Cook for 8 minutes stirring halfway through.
4. Drizzle the nuts with olive oil and salt and shake them well.
5. Cook the nuts for 1 minute.
6. Transfer the cooked nuts ramekins.

Nutrition:
calories 230,
fat 23.9,
fiber 2.4,
carbs 3.9,
protein 3.9

Flax Mozzarella Wraps
Preparation time: 10 minutes
Cooking time: 2 minutes
Servings: 2
Ingredients:

- 1 cucumber
- 1 egg
- 3 oz. flax seeds
- 3 oz. mozzarella, grated
- 1 tablespoon water
- ½ tablespoon butter
- ¼ teaspoon baking soda
- ¼ teaspoon salt

Directions:
1. Crack the egg into a bowl and whisk it.
2. Sprinkle the whisked egg with the flax seeds, grated mozzarella, water, baking soda, and salt.
3. Whisk the mixture.
4. Preheat the air fryer to 360 F.
5. Toss the butter in the air fryer basket and melt it.
6. Separate the egg liquid into 2 servings.
7. Pour the first part of the serving in the air fryer basket.
8. Cook it for 1 minute on one side.

9. Turn over and cook for another minute.
10. Repeat the same steps with the remaining egg mixture.
11. Cut the cucumber into cubes.
12. Separate the cubed cucumber into 2 parts.
13. Place the cucumber cubes in the center of each egg pancake.
14. Wrap the eggs.

Nutrition:
calories 143,
fat 8.4,
fiber 6.2,
carbs 7.3,
protein 8.6

Zucchini Fritters with Cheddar

Preparation time: 10 minutes
Cooking time: 8 minutes
Servings: 7
Ingredients:

- 4 oz. Mozzarella
- 3 oz. Cheddar cheese
- 1 zucchini, grated
- 2 tablespoon dried dill
- 1 tablespoon coconut flour
- 1 tablespoon almond flour
- ¼ teaspoon salt
- 1 teaspoon butter

Directions:

1. Shred the Cheddar and Mozzarella.
2. Combine the grated zucchini with the shredded cheese.
3. Add dried dill and coconut flour.
4. Add almond flour and salt.
5. Stir carefully with a fork.

6. Mix well to combine and leave to marinade for 3 minutes.
7. Preheat the air fryer to 400 F.
8. Melt the butter in the air fryer tray.
9. Make the fritters from the zucchini mixture and put them in the melted butter.
10. Cook the fritters for 5 minutes.
11. Turn the zucchini fritters over and cook for 3 minutes more.

Nutrition:
calories 133,
fat 9.6,
fiber 1.3,
carbs 3.7,
protein 9.1

Keto Almond Buns

Preparation time: 15 minutes
Cooking time: 13 minutes
Servings: 10
Ingredients:

- 1 cup almond flour
- 5 tablespoon sesame seeds
- 1 tablespoon pumpkin seeds, crushed
- 1 teaspoon stevia extract
- ½ tablespoon baking powder
- 1 teaspoon apple cider vinegar
- ¼ teaspoon salt
- ½ cup water, hot
- 4 eggs

Directions:

1. Place the almond flour, sesame seeds, crushed pumpkin

seeds, baking powder, and salt in a large mixing bowl.

2. Then crack the eggs in a separate bowl.

3. Whisk them and add stevia extract and apple cider vinegar.

4. Stir the egg mixture gently.

5. Pour the hot water into the almond flour mixture.

6. Stir and add the whisked egg mixture.

7. Knead the dough until well combined.

8. Preheat the air fryer to 350 F.

9. Cover the air fryer basket with some parchment paper.

10. Make 10 small buns from the dough and put them in the air fryer.

11. Cook the sesame cloud buns for 13 minutes.

12. Check if the buns are cooked. If they require a little more time – cook for 1 minute more.

13. Allow to cool before serving.

Nutrition:
calories 72, fat 5.8, fiber 0.9, carbs 2.3, protein 3.8

Dessert

Brown Muffins
Preparation time: 15 minutes
Cooking time: 10 minutes
Servings: 2
Ingredients:
- 1 egg, beaten
- 1 tablespoon coconut oil, softened
- 2 tablespoons almond flour
- 1 tablespoon cocoa powder
- 1 tablespoon Erythritol
- 1 teaspoon ground cinnamon

Directions:
1. Mix egg with coconut oil, almond flour, cocoa powder, Erythritol, and ground cinnamon.
2. Pour the muffin batter in the muffin molds.
3. Bake the muffins at 375F for 10 minutes.

Nutrition:
calories 141,
fat 12.7,
 fiber 2.2,
carbs 4.1,
protein 4.8

Lime Bars
Preparation Time: 10 minutes
Cooking time: 35 minutes
Servings: 10
Ingredients:
- 3 tablespoons coconut oil, melted
- 3 tablespoons Splenda
- 1 ½ cup coconut flour
- 3 eggs, beaten
- 1 teaspoon lime zest, grated
- 3 tablespoons lime juice

Directions:
1. Cover the air fryer basket bottom with baking paper.
2. Then in the mixing bowl, mix Splenda with coconut flour, eggs, lime zest, and lime juice.
3. Pour the mixture in the air fryer basket and flatten gently.
4. Cook the meal at 350F for 35 minutes.

5. Then cool the cooked meal little and cut into bars.

Nutrition:
calories 144,
fat 7.2,
fiber 7.2,
 carbs 15.7,
protein 4.1

Tender Macadamia Bars
Preparation time: 15 minutes
Cooking time: 30 minutes
Servings: 10
Ingredients:
- 3 tablespoons butter, softened
- 1 teaspoon baking powder
- 1 teaspoon apple cider vinegar
- 1.5 cup coconut flour
- 3 tablespoons swerve
- 1 teaspoon vanilla extract
- 2 eggs, beaten
- 2 oz macadamia nuts, chopped
- Cooking spray

Directions:
1. Spray the air fryer basket with cooking spray.
2. Then mix all remaining ingredients in the mixing bowl and stir until you get a homogenous mixture.
3. Pour the mixture in the air fryer basket and cook at 345F for 30 minutes.
4. When the mixture is cooked, cut it into bars and transfer in the serving plates.

Nutrition:
calories 158, fat 10.4,
fiber 7.7, carbs 13.1,
protein 4

Cinnamon Zucchini Bread
Preparation Time: 10 minutes
Cooking time: 40 minutes
Servings: 12
Ingredients:
- 2 cups coconut flour
- 2 teaspoons baking powder
- ¾ cup Erythritol
- ½ cup coconut oil, melted
- 1 teaspoon apple cider vinegar
- 1 teaspoon vanilla extract
- 3 eggs, beaten
- 1 zucchini, grated
- 1 teaspoon ground cinnamon

Directions:
1. In the mixing bowl, mix coconut flour with baking powder, Erythritol, coconut oil, apple cider vinegar, vanilla extract, eggs, zucchini, and ground cinnamon.
2. Transfer the mixture in the air fryer basket and flatten it in the shape of the bread.
3. Cook the bread at 350F for 40 minutes.

Nutrition:
calories 179,
fat 12.2,
fiber 8.3,
carbs 14.6,
protein 4.3

CHAPTER 5:

March

Lunch

Paprika Eggs
Preparation time: 10 minutes
Cooking time: 17 minutes
Servings: 2
Ingredients:
- 4 eggs
- 1 teaspoon paprika
- 1 tablespoon cream
- 1 tablespoon chives
- ½ teaspoon salt
- 1 teaspoon dried parsley
- 1 teaspoon oregano

Directions:
1. Put the eggs in the air fryer basket and cook them for 17 minutes at 320 F.
2. Meanwhile, combine the cream, salt, dried parsley, and oregano in a shallow bowl.
3. Chop the chives and add to the cream mixture.
4. When the eggs are cooked – place them in the cold water and let them cool.
5. Once cooled, peel the eggs and cut them into halves.
6. Remove the egg yolks and add them to the cream mixture.
7. Mash well with a fork.
8. Then fill the egg whites with the cream-egg yolk mixture.
9. Serve immediately.

Nutrition:
calories 136,
fat 9.3,
fiber 0.8,
carbs 2.1,
protein 11.4

Crunchy Canadian Bacon
Preparation time: 7 minutes
Cooking time: 10 minutes
Servings: 4
Ingredients:
- ½ teaspoon ground thyme
- ½ teaspoon ground coriander
- ¼ teaspoon ground black pepper
- ½ teaspoon salt
- 1 teaspoon cream
- 10 oz. Canadian bacon

Directions:
1. Slice Canadian bacon.
2. Combine the ground thyme, ground coriander, ground black pepper, and salt in the shallow bowl. Shake gently.

3. Then sprinkle the sliced bacon with the spices.
4. Preheat the air fryer to 360 F.
5. Put the Prepared sliced bacon in the air fryer and cook it for 5 minutes.
6. Turn the bacon over and cook it for 5 minutes more.
7. When the bacon is cooked and slightly crunchy remove from the air fryer and serve it with the cream.

Nutrition:
calories 150,
fat 6.7,
fiber 0.1,
carbs 1.9,
protein 19.6

Kale Fritters
Preparation time: 10 minutes
Cooking time: 8 minutes
Servings: 8
Ingredients:
- 12 oz. kale
- 3 oz chive stems
- 1 tablespoon butter
- 1 egg
- 2 tablespoons almond flour
- ½ teaspoon salt
- 1 teaspoon paprika
- 1 tablespoon cream
- 1 teaspoon oil

Directions:
1. Wash the kale carefully and chop it roughly.
2. Place the chopped kale in a blender and blend it until smooth.
3. Dice the chives.
4. Crack the egg in a bowl and whisk it using a hand whisker.
5. Add almond flour, salt, paprika, and cream. Stir it.
6. Then add the diced chives and blended kale.
7. Mix it up until you get well combined fritter dough.
8. Preheat the air fryer to 360 F.
9. Grease the air fryer basket tray with the olive oil.
10. Make 8 medium fritters from the Prepared dough and place them in the air fryer basket tray.
11. Cook the kale fritters for 4 minutes on each side.
12. When the kale fritters are cooked – remove them from the air fryer and chill.

Nutrition:
calories 86,
fat 5.6,
fiber 1.6,
carbs 6.8,
protein 3.6

Keto Almond Bread
Preparation time: 20 minutes
Cooking time: 25 minutes
Servings: 19
Ingredients:
- 1 cup almond flour
- 3 eggs
- ¼ cup butter
- 1 teaspoon baking powder
- ¼ teaspoon salt

Directions:

1. Crack the eggs into a bowl and mix them using a hand mixer.
2. Melt the butter to room temperature.
3. Add the butter to the egg mixture.
4. Add salt, baking powder, and almond flour.
5. Knead the smooth non-sticky dough.
6. Cover the dough with a towel and leave for 10 minutes to rest.
7. Meanwhile, preheat the air fryer to 360 F.
8. Place the dough in the air fryer tin and cook for 10 minutes.
9. Reduce the temperature to 350 F and cook the bread for 15 minutes more.
10. When the time is over – check if the bread is cooked with the help of a toothpick.
11. Transfer the bread to the wooden board and let it chill.

Nutrition:
calories 40,
fat 3.9,
fiber 0.2,
carbs 0.5,
protein 1.2

Tuna Bacon Boats
Preparation time: 10 minutes
Cooking time: 10 minutes
Servings: 4
Ingredients:

- ¼ teaspoon salt
- 6 oz. bacon, sliced
- ¼ teaspoon turmeric
- ½ teaspoon ground black pepper
- 6 oz. tuna
- 1 teaspoon cream
- 4 oz. Parmesan
- 1 teaspoon butter

Directions:

1. Take 4 air fryer ramekins and line with the sliced bacon.
2. Put a small amount of the butter in every ramekin.
3. Combine the salt, turmeric, and ground black pepper together. Mix well.
4. Grate the Parmesan.
5. Chop the tuna and combine it with the spice mixture.
6. Place the chopped tuna in the bacon ramekins.
7. Add the cream and shredded cheese.
8. Preheat the air fryer to 360 F.
9. Put the tuna boats in the air fryer basket and cook for 10 minutes or until crunchy and golden brown.

Nutrition:
calories 411,
fat 28.3,
fiber 0.1,
carbs 1.9,
protein 36.2

Coconut Cookies
Preparation time: 10 minutes
Cooking time: 15 minutes
Servings: 12
Ingredients:

- ½ cup coconut flour

- ½ cup almond flour
- 1/3 teaspoon salt
- 1 teaspoon baking powder
- 1 teaspoon apple cider vinegar
- 4 oz. bacon, cooked, chopped
- 3 tablespoon butter
- 1 tablespoon cream
- 1 egg

Directions:

1. Crack the egg in a bowl and whisk it.
2. Add the baking powder, apple cider vinegar, and cream.
3. Stir it gently and add butter.
4. Add salt, almond flour, and coconut flour.
5. Sprinkle the mixture with the chopped bacon and knead the dough until smooth, soft, and slightly sticky.
6. Preheat the air fryer to 360 F.
7. Cover the air fryer tray with foil.
8. Make 6 medium balls from the Preparationared dough and place the balls in the air fryer basket.
9. Cook the cookies for 15 minutes.
10. Allow to cool before serving.

Nutrition:
calories 182, fat 13.1,
fiber 3.3,
carbs 6.7,
protein 8.1

Cauliflower Chicken Hash

Preparation time: 10 minutes
Cooking time: 14 minutes
Servings: 3
Ingredients:

- 6 oz. cauliflower
- 7 oz. chicken fillet
- 1 tablespoon cream
- 3 tablespoon butter
- 1 teaspoon ground black pepper
- 3 oz chive stems
- 1 green pepper
- 1 tablespoon water

Directions:

1. Chop the cauliflower roughly and put it in a blender.
2. Blend it carefully until you get a cauliflower rice.
3. Chop the chicken fillet into small pieces.
4. Sprinkle the chicken with the ground black pepper and mix to combine.
5. Preheat the air fryer to 380 F.
6. Put the chicken in the air fryer basket tray, add water, cream and cook it for 6 minutes.
7. Reduce the heat of the air fryer to 360 F.
8. Dice the chives and chop the green pepper.
9. Add the cauliflower rice, diced chives, and chopped green pepper.
10. Add the butter and mix well.
11. Cook the dish for 8 minutes.

12. Mix the chicken hash carefully and check if all the ingredients are cooked.
13. Serve the chicken hash immediately.

Nutrition:
calories 261,
fat 16.8,
fiber 2.7,
carbs 7.1,
protein 21

Paprika Chicken Strips

Preparation time: 10 minutes
Cooking time: 12 minutes
Servings: 4
Ingredients:

- 1 teaspoon paprika
- ½ teaspoon ground black pepper
- 1 tablespoon butter
- ½ teaspoon salt
- 1-pound chicken fillet
- 1 tablespoon cream

Directions:

1. Cut the chicken fillet into strips.
2. Sprinkle the chicken with the ground black pepper and salt.
3. Preheat the air fryer to 365 F.
4. Put the butter in the air fryer basket tray and add the chicken strips.
5. Cook the chicken strips for 6 minutes.
6. Turn the chicken strips over and cook them for 5 minutes more.
7. After this, sprinkle the chicken strips with the cream and let them rest for 1 minute.
8. Transfer the cooked chicken strips to serving plates.

Nutrition:
calories 245,
fat 11.5,
fiber 0.3,
carbs 0.6,
protein 33

Eggs in Zucchini Nests

Preparation time: 10 minutes
Cooking time: 7 minutes
Servings: 4
Ingredients:

- 8 oz. zucchini
- 4 eggs
- 4 oz. Cheddar cheese, shredded
- ¼ teaspoon salt
- ½ teaspoon ground black pepper
- ½ teaspoon paprika
- 4 teaspoon butter

Directions:

1. Grate the zucchini.
2. Grease 4 ramekins with butter.
3. Add the grated zucchini to make the shape of the nests.
4. Sprinkle the zucchini nests with the salt, ground black pepper, and paprika.
5. Crack the eggs into the zucchini nests and sprinkle each one with the shredded cheese.

6. Preheat the air fryer to 360 F.
7. Put the ramekins in the air fryer basket and cook for 7 minutes.
8. When the zucchini nests are cooked – let them chill for 2-3 minutes.

Nutrition:
calories 221,
fat 17.7,
fiber 0.8,
carbs 2.9,
protein 13.4

Dinner

Buttered Salmon
Basic Recipe
Preparation Time: 5 minutes
Cooking Time: 10 minutes
Serving: 2
Ingredients:

- 2 salmon fillets (6-oz)
- Salt and ground black pepper, as required
- 1 tbspbutter, melted

Directions:

1. Season each salmon fillet with salt and black pepper and then, coat with the butter. Arrange the salmon fillets onto the greased cooking tray.
2. Arrange the drip pan in the bottom of the Instant Vortex Air Fryer Oven cooking chamber. Select "Air Fry" and then adjust the temperature to 360 °F. Set the time for 10 minutes and press "Start".

3. When the display shows "Add Food" insert the cooking tray in the center position. When the display shows "Turn Food" turn the salmon fillets.
4. When cooking time is complete, remove the tray from the Vortex Oven. Serve hot.

Nutrition:
Calories 276
Carbs 0g
Fat 16.3g
Protein 33.1g

Lemony Salmon
Basic Recipe
Preparation Time: 5 minutes
Cooking Time: 10 minutes
Serving: 2
Ingredients:

- 1 tbsp. offresh lemon juice
- ½ tbsp olive oil
- Salt and ground black pepper, as required
- 1 garlic clove, minced
- ½ tsp. fresh thyme leaves, chopped
- 2 (7-oz) Salmon fillets

Directions:

1. In a bowl, add all ingredients except the salmon and mix well. Add the salmon fillets and coat with the mixture generously.
2. Arrange the salmon fillets onto a lightly greased cooking rack, skin-side down. Arrange the drip pan in the bottom of the Instant Vortex Air Fryer Oven cooking chamber. Select "Air Fry" and then adjust the temperature to 400

°F. Set the time for 10 minutes and press "Start".

3. When the display shows "Add Food" insert the cooking rack in the bottom position. When the display shows "Turn Food" turn the fillets.

4. When the cooking time is complete, remove the tray from the Vortex Oven. Serve hot.

Nutrition:
Calories 297
Carbs 0.8g
Fat 15.8g
Protein 38.7g

Miso Glazed Salmon
Basic Recipe
Preparation Time: 5 minutes
Cooking Time: 10 minutes
Serving: 4
Ingredients:

- 1/3 cup sake
- ¼ cup sugar
- ¼ cup red miso
- 1 tbsplow-sodium soy sauce
- 2 tbsp vegetable oil
- 4 (5-oz) Skinless salmon fillets, (1-inch thick)

Directions:

1. Place the sake, sugar, miso, soy sauce and oil into a bowl and beat until thoroughly combined. Rub the salmon fillets with the mixture generously. In a plastic zip lock bag, place the salmon fillets with any remaining miso mixture.

2. Seal the bag and refrigerate to marinate for about 30 minutes Grease a baking dish that will fit in the Vortex Air Fryer Oven.

Remove the salmon fillets from bag and shake off the excess marinade. Arrange the salmon fillets into the prepared baking dish.

3. Arrange the drip pan in the bottom of the Instant Vortex Air Fryer Oven cooking chamber. Select "Broil" and Set the time for 5 minutes.

4. When the display shows "Add Food" insert the baking dish in the center position.

5. When the display shows "Turn Food" do not turn food. When cooking time is complete, remove the baking dish from the Vortex Oven. Serve hot.

Nutrition:
Calories 335
Carbs 18.3g
Fat 16.6g
Protein 29.8g

Spiced Tilapia
Basic Recipe
Preparation Time: 5 minutes
Cooking Time: 12 minutes
Serving: 2
Ingredients:

- ½ Tsplemon pepper seasoning
- ½ tsp. Garlic powder
- ½ tsp onion powder
- Salt and ground black pepper, as required
- 2 (6-oz) tilapia fillets
- 1 tbsp olive oil

Directions:

1. In a small bowl, mix together the spices, salt and black pepper. Coat the tilapia fillets with oil and then

rub with spice mixture. Arrange the tilapia fillets onto a lightly greased cooking rack, skin-side down.

2. Arrange the drip pan in the bottom of the Instant Vortex Air Fryer Oven cooking chamber. Select "Air Fry" and then adjust the temperature to 360 °F. Set the time for 12 minutes and press "Start".

3. When the display shows "Add Food" insert the cooking rack in the bottom position. When the display shows "Turn Food" turn the fillets.

4. When cooking time is complete, remove the tray from the Vortex Oven. Serve hot.

Nutrition:
Calories 206
Carbs 0.2g
Fat 8.6g
Protein 31.9g

Crispy Tilapia
Basic Recipe
Preparation Time: 5 minutes
Cooking Time: 15 minutes
Serving: 2
Ingredients:

- ¾ cup cornflakes, crushed
- 1 (1-oz.) packet, dry ranch-style dressing mix
- 2½ tbsp vegetable oil
- 2eggs
- 4 (6-oz) tilapia fillets

Directions:

1. In a shallow bowl, beat the eggs. In another bowl, add the cornflakes, ranch dressing, and oil

and mix until a crumbly mixture form. Dip the fish fillets into egg and then, coat with the cornflake mixture.

2. Arrange the tilapia fillets onto the greased cooking tray. Arrange the drip pan in the bottom of the Instant Vortex Air Fryer Oven cooking chamber. Select "Air Fry" and then adjust the temperature to 355 °F. Set the time for 14 minutes and press "Start".

3. When the display shows "Add Food" insert the cooking tray in the center position. When the display shows "Turn Food" turn the tilapia fillets. When cooking time is complete, remove the tray from the Vortex Oven. Serve hot.

Nutrition:
Calories 291
Carbs 4.9g
Fat 14.6g
Protein 34.8g

Simple Haddock
Basic Recipe
Preparation Time: 5 minutes
Cooking Time: 10 minutes
Serving: 2
Ingredients:

- 2 (6-oz) haddock fillets
- 1 tbsp olive oil
- Salt and ground black pepper, as required

Directions:

1. Coat the haddock fillets with oil and then, sprinkle with salt and black pepper. Arrange the haddock fillets onto a greased

cooking rack and spray with cooking spray.

2. Arrange the drip pan in the bottom of the Instant Vortex Air Fryer Oven cooking chamber. Select "Air Fry" and then adjust the temperature to 355 °F. Set the time for 8 minutes and press "Start".

3. When the display shows "Add Food" insert the cooking rack in the center position.

4. When the display shows "Turn Food" do not turn food.

5. When the cooking time is complete, remove the rack from the Vortex Oven. Serve hot.

Nutrition:
Calories 251
Carbs 0g
Fat 8.6g
Protein 41.2g

Fish

Pecan Crusted Fish Fillets
Preparation Time: 10 minutes
Cooking Time: 17 minutes
Servings: 2
Ingredients:

- 2 halibut fillets
- 1/2 lemon juice
- 1 teaspoon garlic, minced
- 1/4 cup parmesan cheese, grated
- 1/4 cup pecans
- 2 tablespoon butter
- Pepper
- Salt
-

Directions:

1. Add pecans, lemon juice, garlic, parmesan cheese, and butter into the food processor and process until completely blended.

2. Place the cooking tray in the air fryer basket. Line air fryer basket with parchment paper.

3. Select Bake mode.

4. Set time to 5 minutes and temperature 400 F then press START.

5. The air fryer display will prompt you to ADD FOOD once the temperature is reached then season fish fillets with pepper and salt and place in the air fryer basket.

6. Spread pecan mixture on top of fish fillets and bake for 12 minutes more.

7. Serve and enjoy.

Nutrition:
Calories 606
Fat 33.5 g
Carbohydrates 3.6 g
Sugar 0.7 g
Protein 71.6 g
Cholesterol 144 mg

Bagel Crust Fish Fillets

Preparation Time: 10 minutes
Cooking Time: 10 minutes
Servings: 4
Ingredients:

- 4 white fish fillets
- 1 tablespoon mayonnaise
- 1 teaspoon lemon pepper seasoning
- 2 tablespoon almond flour
- 1/4 cup bagel seasoning

Directions:

1. In a small bowl, mix together bagel seasoning, almond flour, and lemon pepper seasoning.
2. Brush mayonnaise over fish fillets. Sprinkle seasoning mixture over fish fillets.
3. Place the cooking tray in the air fryer basket. Line air fryer basket with parchment paper.
4. Select Bake mode.
5. Set time to 10 minutes and temperature 400 F then press START.
6. The air fryer display will prompt you to ADD FOOD once the temperature is reached then place fish fillets in the air fryer basket.
7. Serve and enjoy.

Nutrition:
Calories 375
Fat 2.5 g
Carbohydrates 7.2 g
Sugar 1 g
Protein 41.3 g
Cholesterol 120 mg

Meat

Asian Meatballs

Preparation Time: 10 minutes
Cooking Time: 15 minutes
Servings: 4
Ingredients:

- 1 lb ground pork
- 1/2 lime juice
- 2 teaspoon curry paste
- 1 tablespoon Worcestershire sauce
- 1 tablespoon soy sauce
- 1 teaspoon garlic puree
- 1 teaspoon coriander
- 1 teaspoon Chinese spice
- 1 onion, chopped
- Pepper
- Salt

Directions:

1. Add ground meat and remaining ingredients into the large bowl and mix until well combined.
2. Make small meatballs from meat mixture.
3. Select Air Fry mode.
4. Set time to 15 minutes and temperature 350 F then press START.
5. The air fryer display will prompt you to ADD FOOD once the temperature is reached then place meatballs in the air fryer basket.
6. Serve and enjoy.

Nutrition:
Calories 201 Fat 5.8 g
Carbohydrates 4.9 g
Sugar 2.1 g Protein 30.5 g
Cholesterol 83 mg

Spicy Pork Patties

Preparation Time: 10 minutes
Cooking Time: 10 minutes
Servings: 2
Ingredients:

- 1/2 lb ground pork
- 1 tablespoon Cajun seasoning
- 1 egg, lightly beaten
- 1/2 cup almond flour
- Pepper
- Salt

Directions:

1. Add all ingredients into the large bowl and mix until well combined.
2. Make two equal shapes of patties from the meat mixture.
3. Select Air Fry mode.
4. Set time to 10 minutes and temperature 360 F then press START.
5. The air fryer display will prompt you to ADD FOOD once the temperature is reached then place patties in the air fryer basket.
6. Serve and enjoy.

Nutrition:
Calories 234
Fat 9.7 g
Carbohydrates 1.7 g
Sugar 0.4 g
Protein 34 g
Cholesterol 165 mg

Herb Pork Chops

Preparation Time: 10 minutes
Cooking Time: 15 minutes
Servings: 4
Ingredients:

- 4 pork chops
- 2 teaspoon oregano
- 2 teaspoon thyme
- 2 teaspoon sage
- 1 teaspoon garlic powder
- 1 teaspoon paprika
- 1 teaspoon rosemary
- Pepper
- Salt

Directions:

1. Spray pork chops with cooking spray.
2. Mix together garlic powder, paprika, rosemary, oregano, thyme, sage, pepper, and salt and rub over pork chops.
3. Select Air Fry mode.
4. Set time to 15 minutes and temperature 360 F then press START.
5. The air fryer display will prompt you to ADD FOOD once the temperature is reached then place pork chops in the air fryer basket. Turn pork chops halfway through.
6. Serve and enjoy.

Nutrition:
Calories 266 Fat 20.2 g
Carbohydrates 2 g Sugar 0.3 g
Protein 18.4 g
Cholesterol 69 mg

<u>Vegetable</u>

Bell Peppers

Preparation Time: 10 minutes
Cooking Time: 8 minutes
Servings: 3
Ingredients:

- 1 cup red bell peppers, cut into chunks

- 1 cup green bell peppers, cut into chunks
- 1 cup yellow bell peppers, cut into chunks
- 1 teaspoon olive oil
- 1/4 teaspoon garlic powder
- Pepper
- Salt

Directions:

1. Add all ingredients into the large bowl and toss well.
2. Select Air Fry mode.
3. Set time to 8 minutes and temperature 360 F then press START.
4. The air fryer display will prompt you to ADD FOOD once the temperature is reached then add bell peppers in the air fryer basket. Stir halfway through.
5. Serve and enjoy.

Nutrition:
Calories 52
Fat 1.9 g
Carbohydrates 9.2 g
Sugar 6.1 g
Protein 1.2 g
Cholesterol 0 mg

Baby Carrots

Preparation Time: 10 minutes
Cooking Time: 12 minutes
Servings: 4
Ingredients:

- 3 cups baby carrots
- 1 tablespoon olive oil
- Pepper
- Salt

Directions:

1. Add carrots, oil, pepper, and salt into the mixing bowl and toss well.
2. Select Bake mode.
3. Set time to 12 minutes and temperature 390 F then press START.
4. The air fryer display will prompt you to ADD FOOD once the temperature is reached then add baby carrots in the air fryer basket. Stir halfway through.
5. Serve and enjoy.

Nutrition:
Calories 52
Fat 3.6 g
Carbohydrates 5.3 g
Sugar 3 g
Protein 0.4 g
Cholesterol 0 mg

Healthy Roasted Broccoli

Preparation Time: 10 minutes
Cooking Time: 20 minutes
Servings: 6
Ingredients:

- 4 cups broccoli florets
- 3 tablespoon olive oil
- 1/2 teaspoon pepper
- 1/2 teaspoon garlic powder
- 1 teaspoon Italian seasoning
- 1 teaspoon salt

Directions:

1. Add broccoli in a baking dish and drizzle with oil and season with garlic powder, Italian seasoning, pepper, and salt.
2. Select Bake mode.

3. Set time to 20 minutes and temperature 400 F then press START.
4. The air fryer display will prompt you to ADD FOOD once the temperature is reached then place the baking dish in the air fryer basket.
5. Serve and enjoy.

Nutrition:
Calories 84
Fat 7.4 g
Carbohydrates 4.4 g
Sugar 1.2 g
Protein 1.8 g
Cholesterol 1 mg

Snacks

Moroccan Lamb Balls
Preparation time: 15 minutes
Cooking time: 14 minutes
Servings: 6
Ingredients:

- 1 teaspoon cumin seeds
- 1 teaspoon coriander seeds
- 1 garlic clove, sliced
- 12 oz. ground lamb
- 2 tablespoon fresh lemon juice
- 1 egg
- 1 teaspoon dried mint
- 2 tablespoon heavy cream

Directions:
1. Combine the ground lamb and sliced garlic in a bowl.
2. Sprinkle the meat mixture with the coriander seeds and cumin seeds.
3. Coat the ground lamb with the fresh lemon juice and dried mint.
4. Stir the ground lamb mixture with a fork.
5. Crack the egg into the mixture.
6. Stir well.
7. Preheat the air fryer 360 F.
8. Make the meatballs from the lamb mixture and place them in the air fryer.
9. Cook for 8 minutes.
10. Drizzle the lamb balls with the heavy cream and cook for 6 minutes.
11. Place a cocktail stick in every lamb ball and serve them.

Nutrition:
calories 137,
fat 6.9,
fiber 0.1,
carbs 0.7,
protein 17.1

Onion Circles
Preparation time: 15 minutes
Cooking time: 8 minutes
Servings: 10
Ingredients:

- 2 white onions
- ½ teaspoon salt
- ½ cup coconut flour
- ½ teaspoon paprika

- ½ teaspoon ground black pepper
- 1 egg
- 1/3 cup heavy cream
- 1/3 cup almond flour
- 1 tablespoon olive oil

Directions:

1. Peel the onions and slice them roughly.

2. Separate the sliced onions into circles.

3. Crack the egg into a bowl and whisk.

4. Sprinkle the whisked egg with the paprika, salt, ground black pepper, and heavy cream.

5. Whisk well until combined.

6. Preheat the air fryer to 360 F.

7. Coat the onion rings in the almond flour.

8. Dip the onion circles in the whisked egg mixture.

9. Coat the onion circles in the coconut flour.

10. Grease the air fryer basket tray with the olive oil and place the onion circles inside.

11. Cook the onion circles for 8 minutes.

Nutrition:
calories 88,
fat 5.7,
fiber 3.3,
carbs 7.1,
protein 2.5

Scotch Beef Eggs

Preparation time: 15 minutes
Cooking time: 13 minutes
Servings: 6
Ingredients:

- 3 eggs, boiled
- ½ cup coconut flour
- 1 egg
- 16 oz. ground beef
- 1 teaspoon salt
- 1 teaspoon ground black pepper
- 1 teaspoon turmeric
- 1 teaspoon olive oil

Directions:

1. Crack the raw egg in a bowl and whisk it.

2. Peel the boiled eggs.

3. Combine the ground beef with salt, ground black pepper, and turmeric.

4. Mix to combine.

5. Make 3 balls from the ground beef mixture and put the boiled eggs inside to make the round meatballs.

6. Dip the meatballs in the whisked egg.

7. Coat the meatballs in the coconut flour generously.

8. Preheat the air fryer to 370 F.

9. Place the scotch eggs inside and drizzle them with olive oil.

10. Cook the dish for 10 minutes.

11. Increase the temperature to 380 F and cook the dish for 3 minutes more.

12.Allow to cool before serving.

Nutrition:
calories 159,
fat 6.3,
fiber 4.1,
carbs 7.2,
protein 17.8

Turmeric Eggplants

Preparation time: 15 minutes
Cooking time: 8 minutes
Servings: 9
Ingredients:

- 2 eggplants
- 1 tablespoon olive oil
- 1 teaspoon minced garlic
- ½ teaspoon salt
- 1 teaspoon ground turmeric
- 1 teaspoon dried rosemary

Directions:

1. Wash the eggplants carefully and slice into thick circles.
2. Combine the olive oil, minced garlic, salt, ground turmeric, and dried rosemary in a bowl.
3. Mix well.
4. Brush each eggplant circle with the oil mixture.
5. Preheat the air fryer to 400 F.
6. Place the eggplant in the air fryer rack and cook for 5 minutes.
7. Turn the eggplant and cook for 3 minutes more or until soft and golden brown.

Nutrition:
calories 49,
fat 1.5,
fiber 4.7,
carbs 7.5,
protein 1.1

Dessert

Almond Pie

Preparation Time: 10 minutes
Cooking time: 35 minutes
Servings: 8
Ingredients:

- 2 eggs, beaten
- ¾ cup Erythritol
- ¼ cup almond flour
- 2 tablespoons coconut oil, melted
- 1 teaspoon lime zest, grated
- 1 teaspoon baking powder
- 1 teaspoon vanilla extract
- ½ teaspoon apple cider vinegar
- 1 oz almonds, chopped

Directions:

1. Mix all ingredients in the mixing bowl and whisk until smooth.
2. Then pour the mixture in the baking pan and flatten gently.
3. Put the baking pan in the air fryer and cook the pie at 365F for 35 minutes.

Nutrition:
calories 89, fat 7.9,
fiber 0.9, carbs 2,
protein 2

Sweet Cream Cheese Zucchini

Preparation Time: 10 minutes
Cooking time: 15 minutes
Servings: 4
Ingredients:

- 4 teaspoons cream cheese
- 1 zucchini, grated
- 2 tablespoons Erythritol
- ¼ cup heavy cream
- 1 teaspoon butter

Directions:

1. Mix cream cheese with grated zucchini, heavy cream, butter, and Erythritol.
2. Put the mixture in the air fryer basket and flatten gently.
3. Cook the meal at 360F for 15 minutes.

Nutrition:
calories 54,
fat 5,
fiber 0.5,
carbs 1.9,
protein 1

Lemon Custard

Preparation time: 10 minutes
Cooking time: 35 minutes
Servings: 2
Ingredients:

- ½ cup heavy cream
- 1 teaspoon lemon zest, grated
- 1 teaspoon vanilla extract
- 1 tablespoon butter, softened
- 3 eggs, beaten

Directions:

1. Whisk all ingredients in the mixing bowl until smooth.
2. Pour the mixture in the baking pan and transfer in the air fryer basket.

3. Cook the custard at 340F for 35 minutes.

Nutrition:
calories 255,
fat 23.4,
fiber 0.1,
carbs 1.8,
protein 9

Vanilla Pie

Preparation time: 10 minutes
Cooking time: 40 minutes
Servings: 8
Ingredients:

- ½ cup coconut cream
- 3 eggs, beaten
- 1 tablespoon vanilla extract
- 1 teaspoon baking powder
- 3 tablespoons swerve
- 1 cup coconut flour
- 1 tablespoon coconut oil, melted

Directions:

1. Mix coconut cream with eggs, vanilla extract, baking powder, swerve, coconut flour, and coconut oil.
2. Then transfer the mixture in the air fryer basket and flatten it gently.
3. Cook the pie at 355F for 40 minutes.

Nutrition:
calories 139,
fat 8.9,
fiber 5.3,
carbs 9.5,
protein 4.4

CHAPTER 6:

April

Lunch

Cheddar Soufflé with Herbs
Preparation time: 10 minutes
Cooking time: 8 minutes
Servings: 4
Ingredients:

- 5 oz. Cheddar cheese, shredded
- 3 eggs
- 4 tablespoon heavy cream
- 1 tablespoon chives
- 1 tablespoon dill
- 1 teaspoon parsley
- ½ teaspoon ground thyme

Directions:

1. Crack the eggs into a bowl and whisk them carefully.
2. Add the heavy cream and whisk it for 10 seconds more.
3. Add the chives, dill, parsley, and ground thyme.
4. Sprinkle the egg mixture with the shredded cheese and stir it.
5. Transfer the egg mixture into 4 ramekins and place the ramekins in the air fryer basket.
6. Preheat the air fryer to 390 F and cook the soufflé for 8 minutes.
7. Once cooked, chill well.

Nutrition:
calories 244,
fat 20.6,
fiber 0.2,
carbs 1.7,
protein 13.5

Bacon Butter Biscuits
Preparation time: 15 minutes
Cooking time: 10 minutes
Servings: 6
Ingredients:

- 1 egg
- 4 oz. bacon, cooked
- 1 cup almond flour
- ½ teaspoon baking soda
- 1 tablespoon apple cider vinegar
- 3 tablespoon butter
- 4 tablespoon heavy cream
- 1 teaspoon dried oregano

Directions:

1. Crack the egg in a bowl and whisk it.
2. Chop the cooked bacon and add it into the whisked egg.

3. Sprinkle the mixture with baking soda and apple cider vinegar.
4. Add the heavy cream and dried oregano. Stir.
5. Add butter and almond flour.
6. Mix well with a hand mixer.
7. When you get a smooth and liquid batter – the dough is cooked.
8. Preheat the air fryer to 400 F.
9. Pour the batter dough into muffin molds.
10. When the air fryer is heated put the muffin molds in the air fryer basket and cook them for 10 minutes.
11. Chill the muffins to room temperature.

Nutrition:
calories 226, fat 20.5,
fiber 0.6,
carbs 1.8,
protein 9.2

Keto Parmesan Frittata

Preparation time: 10 minutes
Cooking time: 15 minutes
Servings: 6
Ingredients:

- 6 eggs
- 1/3 cup heavy cream
- 5 oz chive stems
- 1 tablespoon butter
- 1 teaspoon salt
- 1 tablespoon dried oregano
- 6 oz. Parmesan
- 1 teaspoon chili pepper

Directions:

1. Crack the eggs into the air fryer basket tray and whisk them with a hand whisker.
2. Chop and dice the chives.
3. Add the vegetables to the egg mixture.
4. Pour the heavy cream.
5. Sprinkle the liquid mixture with the butter, salt, dried oregano, and chili pepper.
6. Shred Parmesan cheese and add it to the mixture too.
7. Sprinkle the mixture with a silicone spatula.
8. Preheat the air fryer to 375 F and cook the frittata for 15 minutes.

Nutrition:
calories 202,
fat 15,
fiber 0.7,
carbs 3.4,
protein 15.1

Chicken Liver Pate

Preparation time: 10 minutes
Cooking time: 10 minutes
Servings: 7
Ingredients:

- 1-pound chicken liver
- 1 teaspoon salt
- 4 tablespoon butter
- 1 cup water
- 1 teaspoon ground black pepper
- 5 oz chive stems
- ½ teaspoon dried cilantro

Directions:

1. Chop the chicken liver roughly and place it in the air fryer basket tray.
2. Dice the chives.
3. Pour the water in the air fryer basket tray and add the diced chives.
4. Preheat the air fryer to 360 F and cook the chicken liver for 10 minutes.
5. Once cooked, strain the chicken liver mixture to discard the liquid.
6. Transfer the chicken liver into a blender.
7. Add the butter, ground black pepper, and dried cilantro.
8. Blend the mixture till you get the pate texture.
9. Transfer the liver pate to a bowl and serve it immediately or keep in the fridge.

Nutrition:
calories 173,
fat 10.8,
fiber 0.4,
carbs 2.2,
protein 16.1

Coconut Pancake Hash

Preparation time: 7 minutes
Cooking time: 9 minutes
Servings: 9
Ingredients:

- 1 teaspoon baking soda
- 1 tablespoon apple cider vinegar
- 1 teaspoon salt
- 1 teaspoon ground ginger
- 1 cup coconut flour
- 5 tablespoon butter
- 1 egg
- ¼ cup heavy cream

Directions:

1. Combine the baking soda, salt, ground ginger, and flour in a bowl.
2. Take a separate bowl and crack in the egg.
3. Add butter and heavy cream.
4. Use a hand mixer and mix well.
5. Combine the dry and liquid mixture together and stir it until smooth.
6. Preheat the air fryer to 400 F.
7. Pour the pancake mixture into the air fryer basket tray.
8. Cook the pancake hash for 4 minutes.
9. Scramble the pancake hash well and keep cooking for 5 minutes more.
10. Transfer to serving plates and serve hot.

Nutrition:
calories 148,
fat 11.3,
fiber 5.3,
carbs 8.7,
protein 3.7

Beef Slices

Preparation time: 10 minutes
Cooking time: 20 minutes
Servings: 6
Ingredients:

- 8 oz. ground pork

- 7 oz. ground beef
- 6 oz chive stems
- 1 egg
- 1 tablespoon almond flour
- 1 tablespoon chives
- 1 teaspoon salt
- 1 teaspoon cayenne pepper
- 1 tablespoon dried oregano
- 1 teaspoon butter
- 1 teaspoon olive oil

Directions:

1. Crack the egg into a large bowl.
2. Add the ground beef and ground pork.
3. Add the almond flour, chives, salt, cayenne pepper, dried oregano, and butter.
4. Dice the chives.
5. Put the diced chives in the ground meat mixture.
6. Use your hands to combine the mixture.
7. Preheat the air fryer to 350 F.
8. Make the meatloaf form from the ground meat mixture.
9. Grease the air fryer basket with the olive oil and place the meatloaf inside.
10. Cook the meatloaf for 20 minutes.
11. Allow the meatloaf to rest for a few minutes.
12. Slice and serve.

Nutrition:
calories 176, fat 2.2,
fiber 1.3, carbs 3.4,
protein 22.2

Dinner

Crispy Haddock
Basic Recipe
Preparation Time: 5 minutes
Cooking Time: 10 minutes
Serving: 3
Ingredients:

- ½ Cup flour
- ½ tsp. Paprika
- 1 egg, beaten
- ¼ cup mayonnaise
- 4 oz salt and vinegar kale chips, crushed finely
- 1 lb haddock fillet cut into 6 pieces

Direction:

1. In a shallow dish, mix together the flour and paprika. In a second shallow dish, add the egg and mayonnaise and beat well. In a third shallow dish, place the crushed kale chips.
2. Coat the fish pieces with flour mixture, then dip into egg mixture and finally coat with the kale chips. Arrange the fish pieces onto 2 cooking trays.
3. Arrange the drip pan in the bottom of the Instant Vortex Air Fryer Oven cooking chamber. Select "Air Fry" and then adjust the temperature to 370 °F. Set the time for 10 minutes and press "Start".
4. When the display shows "Add Food" insert 1 cooking tray in the top position and another in the bottom position.

5. When the display shows "Turn Food" do not turn the food but switch the position of cooking trays. When cooking time is complete, remove the trays from the Vortex Oven. Serve hot.

Nutrition:
Calories 456
Carbs 40.9g
Fat 22.7g
Protein 43.5g

Vinegar Halibut
Basic Recipe
Preparation Time: 5 minutes
Cooking Time: 12 minutes
Serving: 2
Ingredients:
- 2 (5-oz) Halibut fillets
- 1 garlic cloves, minced
- 1 tsp fresh rosemary, minced
- 1 tbsp olive oil
- 1 tbsp red wine vinegar
- 1/8 tsp hot sauce

Directions:
1. In a large resealable bag, add all ingredients. Seal the bag and shale well to mix. Refrigerate to marinate for at least 30 minutes Remove the fish fillets from the bag and shake off the excess marinade. Arrange the halibut fillets onto the greased cooking tray.
2. Arrange the drip pan in the bottom of the Instant Vortex Air Fryer Oven cooking chamber. Select "Bake" and then adjust the temperature to 450 °F. Set the time for 12 minutes and press "Start". When the display shows "Add Food" insert the cooking tray in the center position. When the display shows "Turn Food" turn the halibut fillets. When the cooking time is complete, remove the tray from the Vortex Oven. Serve hot.

Nutrition:
Calories 223
Carbs 1g
Fat 10.4g
Protein 30g

Breaded Cod
Basic Recipe
Preparation Time: 5 minutes
Cooking Time: 10 minutes
Serving: 4
Ingredients:
- 1/3 cup all-purpose flour
- Ground black pepper, as required
- 1 large egg
- 2 tbsp water
- 2/3 cup cornflakes, crushed
- 1 tbsp parmesan cheese, grated
- 1/8 tsp cayenne pepper
- 1 lb. Cod fillets –
- Salt, as required

Directions:
1. In a shallow dish, add the flour and black pepper and mix well. In a second shallow dish, add the egg and water and beat well. In a third shallow dish, add the cornflakes, cheese and cayenne pepper and mix well.
2. Season the cod fillets with salt evenly. Coat the fillets with flour mixture, then dip into egg mixture and finally coat with the cornflake mixture.

3. Arrange the cod fillets onto the greased cooking rack. Arrange the drip pan in the bottom of the Instant Vortex Air Fryer Oven cooking chamber. Select "Air Fry" and then adjust the temperature to 400 °F. Set the time for 10 minutes and press "Start".

4. When the display shows "Add Food" insert the cooking rack in the bottom position. When the display shows "Turn Food" turn the cod fillets. When cooking time is complete, remove the tray from the Vortex Oven. Serve hot.

Nutrition:
Calories 168
Carbs 12.1g
Fat 2.7g
Protein 23.7g

Spicy Catfish
Basic Recipe
Preparation Time: 5 minutes
Cooking Time: 15 minutes
Serving: 4
Ingredients:

- 2 tbsp almond flour polenta
- 2 tsp cajun seasoning
- ½ tsp paprika
- ½ tsp garlic powder
- Salt, as required
- 2 (6-oz) catfish fillets
- 1 tbsp olive oil

Directions:

1. In a bowl, mix together the almond flour, Cajun seasoning, paprika, garlic powder, and salt. Add the catfish fillets and coat

evenly with the mixture. Now, coat each fillet with oil.

2. Arrange the fish fillets onto a greased cooking rack and spray with cooking spray. Arrange the drip pan in the bottom of the Instant Vortex Air Fryer Oven cooking chamber. Select "Air Fry" and then adjust the temperature to 400 °F. Set the timer for 14 minutes and press "Start".

3. When the display shows "Add Food" insert the cooking rack in the center position. When the display shows "Turn Food" turn the fillets.

4. When cooking time is complete, remove the rack from the Vortex Oven. Serve hot.

Nutrition:
Calories 32
Carbs 6.7g
Fat 20.3g
Protein 27.3g

Tuna Burgers
Basic Recipe
Preparation Time: 5 minutes
Cooking Time: 6 minutes
Serving: 4
Ingredients:

- 7 ozcanned tuna
- 1 large egg
- ¼ cup breadcrumbs
- 1 tbsp. Mustard
- ¼ tsp garlic powder
- ¼ tsp onion powder
- ¼ tspcayenne pepper
- Salt and ground black pepper, as required

Directions:

1. Add all the ingredients into a bowl and mix until well combined. Make 4 equal-sized patties from the mixture.
2. Arrange the patties onto a greased cooking rack. Arrange the drip pan in the bottom of the Instant Vortex Air Fryer Oven cooking chamber. Select "Air Fry" and then adjust the temperature to 400 °F. Set the time for 6 minutes and press "Start".
3. When the display shows "Add Food" insert the cooking rack in the center position.
4. When the display shows "Turn Food" turn the burgers.
5. When the cooking time is complete, remove the tray from the Vortex Oven. Serve hot.
6. **Nutrition:**

Calories 151
Carbs 6.3g
Fat 6.4g
Protein 16.4g

Crispy Prawns
Basic Recipe
Preparation Time: 5 minutes
Cooking Time: 10 minutes
Serving: 4
Ingredients:

- 1egg
- ½ lb crushed nacho chips
- 12prawns, peeled and deveined

Directions:

1. In a shallow dish, beat the egg. In another shallow dish, place the crushed nacho chips. Coat the prawn into egg and then roll into nacho chips.
2. Arrange the coated prawns onto 2 cooking trays in a single layer.

Arrange the drip pan in the bottom of the Instant Vortex Air Fryer Oven cooking chamber. Select "Air Fry" and then adjust the temperature to 355 °F. Set the time for 8 minutes and press "Start".

3. When the display shows "Add Food" insert 1 tray in the top position and another in the bottom position. When the display shows "Turn Food" do not turn the food but switch the position of cooking trays. When cooking time is complete, remove the trays from the Vortex Oven. Serve hot.

Nutrition:
Calories 386
Carbs 36.1g
Fat 17g
Protein 21g

Fish

Healthy Lemon Pepper Shrimp
Preparation Time: 10 minutes
Cooking Time: 8 minutes
Servings: 2
Ingredients:

- 12 oz shrimp, peeled and deveined
- 1 lemon, sliced
- 1/4 teaspoon garlic powder
- 1/4 teaspoon paprika
- 1 teaspoon lemon pepper
- 1 lemon juice
- 1/2 tablespoon olive oil

Directions:

1. Toss shrimp with garlic powder, paprika, lemon pepper, lemon juice, and olive oil.
2. Place the cooking tray in the air fryer basket.
3. Select Air Fry mode.
4. Set time to 8 minutes and temperature 400 F then press START.
5. The air fryer display will prompt you to ADD FOOD once the temperature is reached then add shrimp in the air fryer basket. Shake basket halfway through.
6. Serve shrimp with lemon slices.

Nutrition:
Calories 251
Fat 6.7 g
Carbohydrates 6.8 g
Sugar 1.4 g
Protein 39.5 g
Cholesterol 358 mg

Parmesan Shrimp

Preparation Time: 10 minutes
Cooking Time: 12 minutes
Servings: 4
Ingredients:

- 1 lb shrimp, peeled & deveined
- 2 tablespoon parsley, minced
- 2 tablespoon parmesan cheese, grated
- 1/8 teaspoon garlic powder
- 2 tablespoon olive oil
- 1/2 teaspoon pepper
- 1/2 teaspoon salt

Directions:

1. In a mixing bowl, toss shrimp with olive oil. Add remaining ingredients and toss until shrimp is well coated.
2. Place the cooking tray in the air fryer basket.
3. Select Air Fry mode.
4. Set time to 12 minutes and temperature 400 F then press START.
5. The air fryer display will prompt you to ADD FOOD once the temperature is reached then add shrimp in the air fryer basket.
6. Stir shrimp halfway through.
7. Serve and enjoy.

Nutrition:
Calories 205
Fat 9.5 g
Carbohydrates 2.2 g
Sugar 0 g
Protein 26.8 g
Cholesterol 241 mg

Flavorful Tuna Steaks

Preparation Time: 10 minutes
Cooking Time: 4 minutes
Servings: 2
Ingredients:

- 12 tuna steaks, skinless and boneless
- 1/2 teaspoon vinegar
- 1 teaspoon sesame oil
- 1 teaspoon ginger, grated
- 4 tablespoon soy sauce

Directions:

1. Add tuna steaks and remaining ingredients in the zip-lock bag. Seal bag and

place in the refrigerator for 30 minutes.
2. Select Air Fry mode.
3. Set time to 4 minutes and temperature 380 F then press START.
4. The air fryer display will prompt you to ADD FOOD once the temperature is reached then place marinated tuna steaks in the air fryer basket.
5. Serve and enjoy.

Nutrition:
Calories 980
Fat 34.4 g
Carbohydrates 3.1 g
Sugar 0.6 g
Protein 154.7 g
Cholesterol 250 mg

Meat

Spicy Parmesan Pork Chops
Preparation Time: 10 minutes
Cooking Time: 9 minutes
Servings: 2
Ingredients:

- 2 pork chops, boneless
- 1 teaspoon paprika
- 3 tablespoon parmesan cheese, grated
- 1/3 cup almond flour
- 1 teaspoon Cajun seasoning
- 1 teaspoon dried mixed herbs

Directions
1. In a shallow bowl, mix together parmesan cheese, almond flour, paprika, mixed herbs, and Cajun seasoning.

2. Spray pork chops with cooking spray and coat with parmesan cheese.
3. Select Air Fry mode.
4. Set time to 9 minutes and temperature 350 F then press START.
5. The air fryer display will prompt you to ADD FOOD once the temperature is reached then place breaded pork chops in the air fryer basket. Turn pork chops halfway through.
6. Serve and enjoy.

Nutrition:
Calories 359
Fat 27.2 g
Carbohydrates 2.6 g
Sugar 0.3 g
Protein 26.4 g
Cholesterol 85 mg

Moist Pork Chops
Preparation Time: 10 minutes
Cooking Time: 14 minutes
Servings: 2
Ingredients:

- 2 pork chops
- 1 teaspoon paprika
- 1 teaspoon garlic powder
- 1 teaspoon olive oil
- Pepper
- Salt

Directions
1. Brush pork chops with olive oil and season with garlic powder, paprika, pepper, and salt.
2. Select Air Fry mode.
3. Set time to 14 minutes and temperature 360 F then press START.

4. The air fryer display will prompt you to ADD FOOD once the temperature is reached then place pork chops in the air fryer basket. Turn pork chops halfway through.
5. Serve and enjoy.

Nutrition:
Calories 284 Fat 22.4 g
Carbohydrates 1.6 g Sugar 0.5 g
Protein 18.4 g Cholesterol 69 mg

Air Fried Pork Bites

Preparation Time: 10 minutes
Cooking Time: 15 minutes
Servings: 4
Ingredients:

- 1 lb pork belly, cut into 1-inch cubes
- 1 teaspoon soy sauce
- Pepper
- Salt

Directions:
1. In a bowl, toss pork cubes with soy sauce, pepper, and salt.
2. Select Air Fry mode.
3. Set time to 15 minutes and temperature 400 F then press START.
4. The air fryer display will prompt you to ADD FOOD once the temperature is reached then place pork cubes in the air fryer basket.
5. Serve and enjoy.

Nutrition:
Calories 524
Fat 30.5 g
Carbohydrates 0.1 g
Sugar 0 g
Protein 52.4 g
Cholesterol 131 mg

Snacks

Creamy Cauliflower Florets

Preparation time: 15 minutes
Cooking time: 16 minutes
Servings: 8
Ingredients:

- 18 oz. cauliflower
- 1 cup heavy cream
- 1 teaspoon salt
- ½ teaspoon ground black pepper
- 1 teaspoon turmeric
- 1 egg
- 2 tablespoons almond flour
- 1 teaspoon oregano
- ½ tablespoon olive oil

Directions:
1. Wash the cauliflower carefully and separate it into medium florets.
2. Crack the egg in a large bowl and whisk.
3. Add salt, ground black pepper, turmeric, almond flour, and oregano.
4. Whisk the mixture until you get a smooth batter.
5. Coat the cauliflower florets with the heavy cream batter.
6. Preheat the air fryer to 360 F.
7. Place the coated cauliflower in the air fryer basket tray.
8. Cook for 12 minutes.

9. Increase the temperature to 390 F and cook for 4 minutes more.

Nutrition:
calories 125,
fat 10.6,
fiber 2.5,
carbs 5.7,
protein 3.8

Zucchini Egg Fritters

Preparation time: 10 minutes
Cooking time: 10 minutes
Servings: 7
Ingredients:

- 1 zucchini, grated
- 1 egg
- 4 tablespoons coconut flour
- ½ teaspoon salt
- ½ tablespoon paprika
- 1 teaspoon butter
- 1 oz chive stems
- ½ teaspoon chili flakes

Directions:

1. Place the grated zucchini in a large mixing bowl.
2. Crack the egg in the zucchini.
3. Then add coconut flour, salt, paprika, diced chives, and chili flakes.
4. Gently mix.
5. Preheat the air fryer to 365 F.
6. Put the butter in the air fryer basket tray and melt it.
7. Make small fritters using a spoon and place them in the melted butter.
8. Cook the fritters for 5 minutes on each side.

9. Chill before serving.

Nutrition:
calories 38,
fat 1.7,
fiber 2.3,
carbs 4.5,
protein 1.8

Chili Chicken Bites

Preparation time: 15 minutes
Cooking time: 15 minutes
Servings: 8
Ingredients:

- 1-pound chicken fillet
- 1 teaspoon chili flakes
- 1 teaspoon turmeric
- 1 teaspoon paprika
- ½ teaspoon curry powder
- ½ cup heavy cream
- 2 tablespoons almond flour
- 1 teaspoon olive oil

Directions:

1. Chop the chicken fillet into 8 cubes.
2. Place the chicken cubes in a large bowl.
3. Sprinkle the meat with the chili flakes, turmeric, paprika, and curry powder.
4. Mix well using your hands.
5. Combine the heavy cream and almond flour in a separate bowl.
6. Whisk well.
7. Preheat the air fryer to 365 F.
8. Place the chicken cubes in the air fryer rack and drizzle them with olive oil.

9. Cook the chicken for 15 minutes.

Nutrition:

calories 151,

fat 8.5,

fiber 0.4,

 carbs 1,

protein 17

Broccoli Coconut Loaf

Preparation Time: 10 minutes

Cooking Time: 30 minutes

Serve: 5

Ingredients:

- 5 eggs, lightly beaten
- 3/4 cup broccoli florets, chopped
- 1 cup cheddar cheese, shredded
- 2 tsp baking powder
- 3 1/1 tbsp coconut flour
- 1 tsp salt

Directions:

1. Add all ingredients into the bowl and mix well.
2. Pour egg mixture into the greased loaf pan.
3. Select BAKE mode, then set the temperature to 350 F and the time to 30 minutes, then press start.

4. When the display shows Add Food then place the loaf pan in the vortex plus air fryer oven.
5. Slice and serve.

Nutrition:

Calories 209

Fat 13.5 g

Carbohydrates 8.9 g

Sugar 1.5 g

Protein 13.2 g

Cholesterol 187 mg

<u>Vegetable</u>

Asian Green Beans

Preparation Time: 10 minutes
Cooking Time: 10 minutes
Servings: 2
Ingredients:

- 8 oz green beans, trimmed and cut in half
- 1 tablespoon tamari
- 1 teaspoon sesame oil

Directions:

1. Add all ingredients into the large bowl and toss well.
2. Select Air Fry mode.
3. Set time to 10 minutes and temperature 350 F then press START.
4. The air fryer display will prompt you to ADD FOOD

once the temperature is reached then add green beans in the air fryer basket. Stir halfway through.

5. Serve and enjoy.

Nutrition:

Calories 61 Fat 2.4 g Carbohydrates 8.6 g Sugar 1.7 g Protein 3 g Cholesterol 0 mg

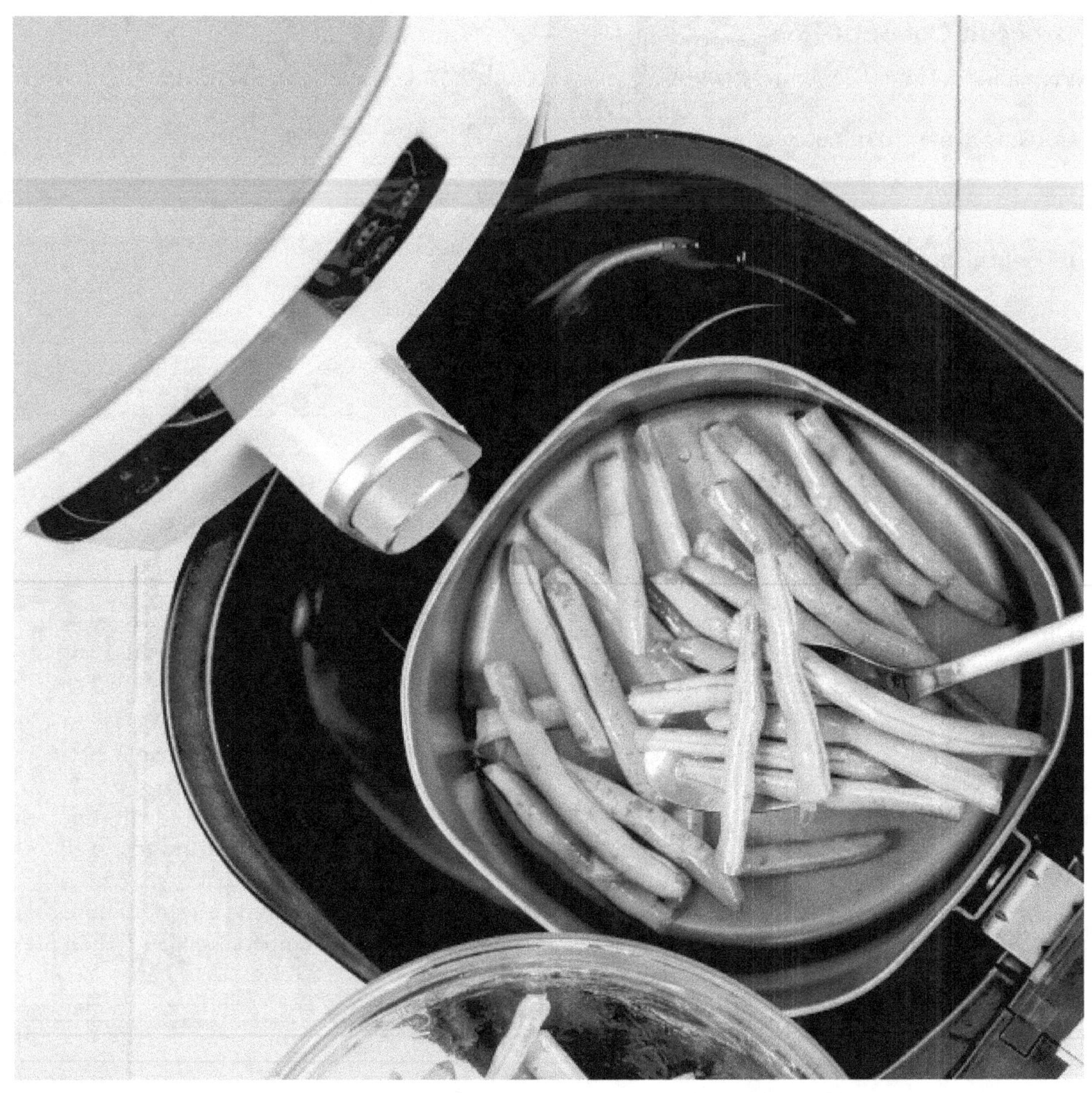

Roasted Veggies

Preparation Time: 10 minutes
Cooking Time: 30 minutes
Servings: 6
Ingredients:

- 1 bell pepper, cut into strips
- 2 zucchini, sliced
- 1 eggplant, sliced
- 1 onion, sliced
- 5 fresh basil leaves, sliced
- 2 teaspoon Italian seasoning
- 2 tablespoon olive oil
- Pepper
- Salt

Directions:

1. Add all ingredients except basil leaves into the mixing bowl and toss well.
2. Select Roast mode.
3. Set time to 30 minutes and temperature 400 F then press START.
4. The air fryer display will prompt you to ADD FOOD once the temperature is reached then place vegetable mixture in the air fryer basket. Stir halfway through.
5. Garnish with basil and serve.

Nutrition:
Calories 95
Fat 5.5 g
Carbohydrates 11.7 g
Sugar 6.4 g
Protein 2.3 g
Cholesterol 1 mg

Cooking Time: 20 minutes
Servings: 6
Ingredients:

- 1 lb fresh spinach
- 1 tablespoon onion, minced
- 8 oz cream cheese
- 6 oz gouda cheese, shredded
- 1 teaspoon garlic powder
- Pepper
- Salt

Directions:

1. Spray a large pan with cooking spray and heat over medium heat.
2. Add spinach to the pan and cook until wilted.
3. Add cream cheese, garlic powder, and onion and stir until cheese is melted.
4. Remove pan from heat and add Gouda cheese and season with pepper and salt.
5. Transfer spinach mixture into the greased baking dish.
6. Select Bake mode.
7. Set time to 20 minutes and temperature 400 F then press START.
8. The air fryer display will prompt you to ADD FOOD once the temperature is reached then place the baking dish in the air fryer basket.
9. Serve and enjoy.

Nutrition:
Calories 253 Fat 21.3 g
Carbohydrates 4.9 g Sugar 1.2 g
Protein 12.2 g Cholesterol 74 mg

Creamy Spinach

Preparation Time: 10 minutes

Broccoli Fritters

Preparation Time: 10 minutes
Cooking Time: 30 minutes
Servings: 4
Ingredients:

- 2 eggs, lightly beaten
- 2 garlic cloves, minced
- 3 cups broccoli florets, steam & chopped
- 1 cup cheddar cheese, shredded
- 1 cup mozzarella cheese, shredded
- 1/4 cup almond flour
- Pepper
- Salt

Directions:

1. Add all ingredients into the large bowl and mix until well combined.
2. Make patties from the broccoli mixture.
3. Select Bake mode.
4. Set time to 30 minutes and temperature 375 F then press START.
5. The air fryer display will prompt you to ADD FOOD once the temperature is reached then place broccoli patties in the air fryer basket.
6. Serve and enjoy.

Nutrition:
Calories 201
Fat 13.9 g
Carbohydrates 6.2 g
Sugar 1.6 g
Protein 14.2 g
Cholesterol 115 mg

Dessert

Poppy Seeds Muffins

Preparation time: 10 minutes
Cooking time: 10 minutes
Servings: 5
Ingredients:

- 5 tablespoons coconut oil, softened
- 1 egg, beaten
- 1 teaspoon vanilla extract
- 1 tablespoon poppy seeds
- 1 teaspoon baking powder
- 2 tablespoons Erythritol
- 1 cup coconut flour

Directions:

1. In the mixing bowl, mix coconut oil with egg, vanilla extract, poppy seeds, baking powder, Erythritol, and coconut flour.
2. When the mixture is homogenous, pour it in the muffin molds and transfer it in the air fryer basket.
3. Cook the muffins for 10 minutes at 365F.

Nutrition:
calories 239,
fat 17.7,
fiber 9.8,
carbs 17.1,
protein 4.6

Raspberry Tart

Preparation Time: 5 minutes
Cooking time: 20 minutes
Servings: 8
Ingredients:

- 5 egg whites
- 1/3 cup Erythritol
- 1.5 cup coconut flour

- 1 teaspoon lime zest, grated
- 1 teaspoon baking powder
- 1/3 cup coconut oil, melted
- 3 oz raspberries
- Cooking spray

Directions:

1. Mix eggs with Erythritol, coconut flour, lime zest, baking powder, and coconut oil.
2. Whisk the mixture until smooth.
3. Then spray the air fryer basket with cooking spray and pour the batter inside.
4. Top the batter with raspberries and cook at 360F for 20 minutes.

Nutrition:

calories 96,
fat 9.2,
fiber 0.8,
carbs 1.9,
protein 2.4

Almond Donuts

Preparation Time: 15 minutes
Cooking time: 14 minutes
Servings: 6
Ingredients:

- 8 ounces almond flour
- 2 tablespoons Erythritol
- 1 egg, beaten
- 2 tablespoons almond butter, softened
- 4 ounces heavy cream
- 1 teaspoon baking powder

Directions:

1. In the mixing bowl, mix almond flour, Erythritol, egg, almond butter, heavy cream, and baking powder. Knead the dough.

2. Roll up the dough and make the donuts with the help of the cutter.
3. Put the donuts in the air fryer basket and cook at 365F for 7 minutes per side.

Nutrition:

calories 323,
fat 29.4,
fiber 4.6,
carbs 10,
protein 10.5

Nutmeg Donuts

Preparation time: 20 minutes
Cooking time: 6 minutes
Servings: 4
Ingredients:

- 1 teaspoon ground nutmeg
- ½ teaspoon baking powder
- ½ cup almond flour
- 1 tablespoon Swerve
- 1 egg, beaten
- 1 tablespoon coconut oil, softened
- Cooking spray

Directions:

1. Spray the air fryer basket with cooking spray from inside.
2. Then mix all remaining ingredients and knead the dough.
3. Make the donuts from the dough and put them in the air fryer.
4. Cook the donuts at 390F for 3 minutes per side.

Nutrition:

calories 69,
fat 6.4,
fiber 0.5,
carbs 1.4,
protein 2.2

CHAPTER 7:

May

Lunch

Egg-Beef Rolls
Preparation time: 15 minutes
Cooking time: 8 minutes
Servings: 6
Ingredients:

- ½ cup almond flour
- ¼ cup water
- 1 teaspoon salt
- 1 egg
- 7 oz. ground beef
- 1 teaspoon paprika
- 1 teaspoon ground black pepper
- 1 tablespoon olive oil

Directions:

1. Boil the water in a small saucepan.
2. Combine the almond flour with salt and stir.
3. Add the boiling water and whisk carefully until the mixture is combined.
4. Knead the dough until smooth.
5. Leave to one side.
6. Combine the ground beef with the paprika and ground black pepper.
7. Mix well and transfer to a pan.
8. Fry the meat mixture for 5 minutes on a medium heat. Stir frequently.
9. Crack the egg into the meat mixture and scramble.
10. Cook the mixture for 4 minutes more.
11. Roll the dough and cut it into 6 squares.
12. Put the ground beef mixture in every square.
13. Roll the squares to make the dough sticks.
14. Sprinkle the dough sticks with olive oil.
15. Put the dough sticks in the air fryer basket.
16. Preheat the air fryer to 350 F and add the egg-meat rolls.
17. Cook the dish for 8 minutes.
18. When the egg-meat rolls are cooked transfer them directly to serving plates.

Nutrition:
calories 150,
fat 9.6,
fiber 1.2,
carbs 2.5,
protein 13

Paprika Egg Rolls

Preparation time: 10 minutes
Cooking time: 8 minutes
Servings: 8
Ingredients:

- 6 tablespoon coconut flour
- ½ teaspoon salt
- 1 teaspoon paprika
- 1 teaspoon butter
- 4 eggs
- 1 teaspoon chives
- 1 tablespoon olive oil
- 2 tablespoon water, boiled, hot

Directions:

1. Put the coconut flour in a bowl.
2. Add salt and hot boiled water.
3. Mix well and knead the dough.
4. Leave the dough to rest.
5. Crack the eggs into another bowl.
6. Add chives and paprika.
7. Whisk with a hand whisker.
8. Melt the butter in a pan.
9. Pour the egg mixture into the pan and form a thin omelet.
10. Cook the omelet for 1 minute on each side.
11. Remove the omelet and roughly chop.
12. Roll the Preparationared dough and cut it into 4 squares.
13. Put the chopped eggs in the dough squares and roll them into four tubes.
14. Brush the egg rolls with olive oil.
15. Preheat the air fryer to 355 F.
16. Put the egg rolls in the basket and place in the air fryer.
17. Cook the dish for 8 minutes or until golden brown.
18. Serve hot.

Nutrition:
calories 74,
fat 5,
fiber 2.3,
carbs 4.1,
protein 36

Chicken-Pork Sausages

Preparation time: 15 minutes
Cooking time: 12 minutes
Servings: 6
Ingredients:

- 7 oz. ground chicken
- 7 oz. ground pork
- 1 teaspoon minced garlic
- 1 teaspoon salt
- ½ teaspoon nutmeg
- 1 teaspoon olive oil
- 1 tablespoon almond flour
- 1 egg
- 1 teaspoon chili flakes
- 1 teaspoon ground coriander

Directions:

1. Combine the ground chicken and ground pork together in a bowl.
2. Crack the egg into the mixture.

3. Mix well with a spoon.

4. Sprinkle the mixture with minced garlic, salt, nutmeg, almond flour, chili flakes, and ground coriander.

5. Combine well.

6. Preheat the air fryer to 360 F.

7. Make medium sausages from the mixture.

8. Spray the air fryer basket tray with olive oil.

9. Put the sausages in the air fryer basket and place in the air fryer.

10. Cook for 6 minutes.

11. Turn the sausages over and cook for 6 minutes more.

12. Allow the sausages to cool a little.

13. Serve.

Nutrition:
calories 156,
fat 7.5,
fiber 0.6,
carbs 1.3,
protein 20.2

Almond Blackberry Muffins

Preparation time: 15 minutes
Cooking time: 10 minutes
Servings: 5
Ingredients:

- 1 teaspoon apple cider vinegar
- 1 cup almond flour
- 4 tablespoon butter
- 6 tablespoon almond milk
- 1 teaspoon baking soda
- 3 oz. blackberry
- ½ teaspoon salt
- 3 teaspoon stevia
- 1 teaspoon vanilla extract

Directions:

1. Put the almond flour in a mixing bowl.
2. Add baking soda, salt, stevia, and vanilla extract.
3. Add butter, almond milk, and apple cider vinegar.
4. Crush the blackberries gently and add into the almond flour mixture.
5. Stir carefully with a fork until well combined.
6. Leave the mixture to one side for 5 minutes.
7. Meanwhile, preheat the air fryer to 400 F.
8. Preparationare the muffin molds.
9. Pour the dough in the muffin molds filling half way.
10. Put the muffing molds in the air fryer basket. Close the air fryer.
11. Cook the muffins for 10 minutes.
12. Remove the muffins from the air fryer basket.
13. Chill them until warm.
14. Serve.

Nutrition:
calories 165,
fat 16.4,
fiber 1.9,
carbs 4,
protein 2

Beef Cheddar Chili

Preparation time: 10 minutes
Cooking time: 10 minutes
Servings: 4
Ingredients:

- 3 oz chive stems
- 8 oz. ground beef
- 1 tablespoon dried dill
- 1 teaspoon dried oregano
- 1 teaspoon dried cilantro
- 1 teaspoon dried parsley
- 6 oz. Cheddar cheese, shredded
- 1 teaspoon mustard
- 1 tablespoon butter

Directions:

1. Dice the chives and combine it with the ground beef in a bowl.
2. Sprinkle the mixture with dried dill, dried oregano, dried cilantro, and dried parsley.
3. Then add mustard and butter.
4. Mix well.
5. Preheat the air fryer to 380 F.
6. Put the ground beef mixture in the air fryer basket tray and cook the chili for 9 minutes.
7. Stir it carefully after 6 minutes of cooking.
8. When the chili is cooked – sprinkle with the shredded cheese and stir carefully.
9. Cook the dish for 1 minute more.
10. Then mix the chili mixture carefully again and transfer to bowls.

Nutrition:
calories 315,
fat 20.8,
fiber 0.7,
carbs 2.9,
protein 28.4

Cheddar Chicken Casserole

Preparation time: 15 minutes
Cooking time: 18 minutes
Servings: 6
Ingredients:

- 9 oz. ground chicken
- 5 oz. bacon, sliced
- 3 oz chive stems
- 1 teaspoon salt
- ½ teaspoon ground black pepper
- 1 teaspoon paprika
- 1 teaspoon turmeric
- 6 oz. Cheddar cheese
- 1 egg
- ½ cup cream
- 1 tablespoon almond flour
- 1 tablespoon butter

Directions:

1. Take the air fryer basket tray and grease it with butter.
2. Put the ground chicken in a large bowl and add salt and ground black pepper.
3. Add paprika and turmeric and stir the mixture well with a spoon.
4. Shred the Cheddar cheese.

5. Beat the egg in the ground chicken mixture until it is well combined.
6. Then whisk together the cream and almond flour.
7. Dice the chives.
8. Place the ground chicken in the bottom of the air fryer tray.
9. Sprinkle the ground chicken with the diced chives and cream mixture.
10. Make a layer from the shredded cheese and sliced bacon.
11. Preheat the air fryer to 380 F.
12. Cook the chicken casserole for 18 minutes.
13. When the casserole is cooked – let it chill briefly.

Nutrition:
calories 396,
fat 28.6,
fiber 1,
carbs 3.8,
protein 30.4

Dinner

Prawns in Butter Sauce
Basic Recipe
Preparation Time: 5 minutes
Cooking Time: 6 minutes
Serving: 2
Ingredients:

½ lb. Peeled and deveined large prawns
1 large garlic clove, minced
1 tbspbutter melted
1 tsp fresh lemon zest grated

Directions:

1. Add all the ingredients into a bowl and toss to coat well. Set aside at room temperature for about 30 minutes.
2. Arrange the prawn mixture into a baking dish that will fit in the Vortex Air Fryer Oven. Arrange the drip pan in the bottom of the Instant Vortex Air Fryer Oven cooking chamber. Select "Bake" and then adjust the temperature to 450 °F.
3. Set the time for 6 minutes and press "Start".
4. When the display shows "Add Food" insert the baking dish in the center position. When cooking time is complete, remove the baking dish from the Vortex Oven. When the display shows "Turn Food" do not turn food.
5. When cooking time is complete, remove the baking dish from the Vortex Oven. Serve hot.

Nutrition:
Calories 189
Carbs 2.4g
Fat 7.7g
Protein 26g

Air Fried Chicken Tenderloin
Basic Recipe
Preparation Time: 5 minutes
Cooking Time: 15 minutes
Serving: 8
Ingredients:

- ½ cup almond flour
- 1 egg, beaten
- 2 tablespoons coconut oil
- 8 chicken tenderloins

- Salt and pepper to taste

Directions:

1. Preheat the air fryer for 5 minutes Season the chicken tenderloin with salt and pepper to taste.
2. Soak in beaten eggs then dredge in almond flour. Place in the air fryer and brush with coconut oil.
3. Cook for 15 minutes at 3750F.
4. Halfway through the cooking time, give the fryer basket a shake to cook evenly.

Nutrition:
Calories 130.3
Carbs 0.7g
Protein 8.7 g
Fat 10.3 g

Almond Flour Battered Chicken Cordon Bleu

Basic Recipe
Preparation Time: 5 minutes
Cooking Time: 30 minutes
Serving: 2
Ingredients:

- ¼ cup almond flour
- 1 slice cheddar cheese
- 1 slice of ham
- 1 small egg, beaten
- 1 teaspoon parsley
- 2 chicken breasts, butterflied
- Salt and pepper to taste

Directions:

1. Season the chicken with parsley, salt and pepper to taste.
2. Place the cheese and ham in the middle of the chicken and roll. Secure with toothpick.
3. Soak the rolled-up chicken in egg and dredge in almond flour.

4. Place in the air fryer.
5. Cook for 30 minutes at 3500F.

Nutrition:
Calories 1142
Carbs 5.5g
Protein 79.4g
Fat 89.1g

Almond Flour Coco-Milk Battered Chicken

Basic Recipe
Preparation Time: 5 minutes
Cooking Time: 30 minutes
Serving: 4
Ingredients:

- ¼ cup coconut milk
- ½ cup almond flour
- 1 ½ tablespoons old bay Cajun seasoning
- 1 egg, beaten
- 4 small chicken thighs
- Salt and pepper to taste

Directions:

1. Preheat the air fryer for 5 minutes
2. Mix the egg and coconut milk in a bowl.
3. Soak the chicken thighs in the beaten egg mixture.
4. In a mixing bowl, combine the almond flour, Cajun seasoning, salt and pepper.
5. Dredge the chicken thighs in the almond flour mixture.
6. Place in the air fryer basket.
7. Cook for 30 minutes at 3500F.

Nutrition:
Calories 590
Carbs3.2g
Protein 32.5 g
Fat 38.6g

Bacon 'n Egg-Substitute Bake

Basic Recipe
Preparation Time: 5 minutes
Cooking Time: 30 minutes
Serving: 4
Ingredients:

- 1 (6 ounce) package Canadian bacon, quartered
- 1/2 cup 2% milk
- 1/4 teaspoon ground mustard
- 1/4 teaspoon salt
- 2 cups shredded Cheddar-Monterey Jack cheese blend
- 3/4 cup and 2 tablespoons egg substitute (such as Egg Beaters® Southwestern Style)
- 4 frozen hash brown patties

Directions:

1. Lightly grease baking pan of air fryer with cooking spray.
2. Evenly spread hash brown patties on bottom of pan. Top evenly with bacon and then followed by cheese.
3. In a bowl, whisk well mustard, salt, milk, and egg substitute. Pour over bacon mixture.
4. Cover air fryer baking pan with foil.
5. Preheat air fryer to 330oF.
6. Cook for another 20 minutes, remove foil and continue cooking for another 15 minutes or until eggs are set.
7. Serve and enjoy.

Nutrition:
Calories 459
Carbs 21.0g
Protein 29.4g
Fat 28.5g

Baked Cauliflower Rice, Black Bean and Cheese

Intermediate Recipe
Preparation Time: 5 minutes
Cooking Time: 1 hour
Serving: 4
Ingredients:

- 1 cooked skinless boneless chicken breast halves, chopped
- 1 cup shredded Swiss cheese
- 1/2 (15 ounce) can black beans, Dry out
- 1/2 (4 ounce) can diced green chili peppers, Dry out
- 1/2 cup vegetable broth
- 1/2 medium zucchini, thinly sliced
- 1/4 cup sliced mushrooms
- 1/4 teaspoon cumin
- 1-1/2 teaspoons olive oil
- 2 tablespoons and 2 teaspoons diced onion
- 3 tablespoons cauliflower rice
- 3 tablespoons shredded carrots
- Ground cayenne pepper to taste
- Salt to taste

Directions:

1. Lightly grease baking pan of air fryer with cooking spray. Add cauliflower rice and broth. Cover pan with foil cook for 10 minutes at 390oF. Lower heat to 300oF and cauliflower rice. Cook for another 10 minutes Let it stand for 10 minutes and transfer to a bowl and set aside.
2. Add oil to same baking pan. Stir in onion and cook for 5 minutes at 330oF.

3. Stir in mushrooms, chicken, and zucchini. Mix well and cook for 5 minutes

4. Stir in cayenne pepper, salt, and cumin. Mix well and cook for another 2 minutes

5. Stir in ½ of the Swiss cheese, carrots, chilies, beans, and cauliflower rice. Toss well to mix. Evenly spread in pan. Top with remaining cheese.

6. Cover pan with foil.

7. Cook for 15 minutes at 390oF and then remove foil and cook for another 5 to 10 minutes or until tops are lightly browned.

8. Serve and enjoy.

Nutrition:
Calories 337
Carbs 11.5g
Protein 25.3g
Fat 21.0g

Fish

Easy Air Fryer Scallops
Preparation Time: 10 minutes
Cooking Time: 4 minutes
Servings: 2
Ingredients:

- 8 scallops
- 1 tablespoon olive oil
- Pepper
- Salt

Directions:

1. Brush scallops with olive oil and season with pepper and salt.

2. Place the cooking tray in the air fryer basket.

3. Select Air Fry mode.

4. Set time to 2 minutes and temperature 390 F then press START.

5. The air fryer display will prompt you to ADD FOOD once the temperature is reached then add scallops in the air fryer basket.

6. Turn scallops and air fry for 2 minutes more.

7. Serve and enjoy.

Nutrition:
Calories 166
Fat 7.9 g
Carbohydrates 2.9 g
Sugar 0 g
Protein 20.2 g
Cholesterol 40 mg

Pesto Scallops
Preparation Time: 10 minutes
Cooking Time: 7 minutes
Servings: 4
Ingredients:

- 1 lb sea scallops
- 2 teaspoon garlic, minced
- 3 tablespoon heavy cream
- 1/4 cup basil pesto
- 1 tablespoon olive oil
- 1/2 teaspoon pepper
- 1 teaspoon salt

Directions:

1. In a small pan, mix together oil, cream, garlic, pesto, pepper, and salt, and simmer for 2-3 minutes.

2. Select Air Fry mode.

3. Set time to 5 minutes and temperature 320 F then press START.

4. The air fryer display will prompt you to ADD FOOD once the temperature is reached then add scallops in the air fryer basket.
5. Turn scallops and after 3 minutes.
6. Transfer scallops into the mixing bowl.
7. Pour pesto sauce over scallops and serve.

Nutrition:
Calories 172
Fat 8.6 g
Carbohydrates 3.7 g
Sugar 0 g
Protein 19.4 g
Cholesterol 53 mg

Meat

Beef Kebabs
Preparation Time: 10 minutes
Cooking Time: 15 minutes
Servings: 4
Ingredients:
- 1 lb ground beef
- 1/2 cup onion, minced
- 1/4 teaspoon ground cinnamon
- 1/4 teaspoon ground cardamom
- 1/2 teaspoon cayenne
- 1/2 teaspoon turmeric
- 1/2 tablespoon ginger paste
- 1/2 tablespoon garlic paste
- 1/4 cup cilantro, chopped
- 1 teaspoon salt

Directions:
1. Add meat and remaining ingredients into the large bowl and mix until well combined.

2. Make sausage shape kebabs.
3. Select Bake mode.
4. Set time to 15 minutes and temperature 350 F then press START.
5. The air fryer display will prompt you to ADD FOOD once the temperature is reached then place kebabs in the air fryer basket.
6. Serve and enjoy.

Nutrition:
Calories 223
Fat 7.2 g
Carbohydrates 2.7 g
Sugar 0.7 g
Protein 34.8 g
Cholesterol 101 mg

Steak Tips
Preparation Time: 10 minutes
Cooking Time: 5 minutes
Servings: 3
Ingredients:
- 1 lb steak, cut into cubes
- 1 teaspoon olive oil
- 1 teaspoon Montreal steak seasoning
- Pepper
- Salt

Directions:
1. In a bowl, add steak cubes and remaining ingredients and toss well.
2. Select Air Fry mode.
3. Set time to 5 minutes and temperature 400 F then press START.
4. The air fryer display will prompt you to ADD FOOD once the temperature is reached then place steak cubes in the air fryer basket.

5. Serve and enjoy.

Nutrition:
Calories 317 Fat 9.1 g
Carbohydrates 0 g
Sugar 0 g Protein 54.6 g
Cholesterol 136 mg

Rosemary Beef Tips

Preparation Time: 10 minutes
Cooking Time: 12 minutes
Servings: 4
Ingredients:

- 1 lb steak, cut into 1-inch cubes
- 1 teaspoon paprika
- 2 teaspoon onion powder
- 1 teaspoon garlic powder
- 2 tablespoon coconut aminos
- 2 teaspoon rosemary, crushed
- Pepper
- Salt

Directions:

1. Add meat and remaining ingredients into the mixing bowl and mix well and let it sit for 5 minutes.
2. Select Air Fry mode.
3. Set time to 12 minutes and temperature 380 F then press START.
4. The air fryer display will prompt you to ADD FOOD once the temperature is reached then place steak cubes in the air fryer basket. Stir halfway through.
5. Serve and enjoy.

Nutrition:
Calories 243 Fat 5.9 g
Carbohydrates 3.7 g
Sugar 0.7 g
Protein 41.3 g
Cholesterol 102 mg

Vegetable

Crispy Brussels Sprouts

Preparation Time: 10 minutes
Cooking Time: 14 minutes
Servings: 2
Ingredients:

- 1/2 lb Brussels sprouts, trimmed and halved
- 1/2 teaspoon chili powder
- 1/2 tablespoon olive oil
- Pepper
- Salt

Directions:

1. Add all ingredients into the large bowl and toss well.
2. Select Air Fry mode.
3. Set time to 14 minutes and temperature 350 F then press START.
4. The air fryer display will prompt you to ADD FOOD once the temperature is reached then add brussels sprouts in the air fryer basket.
5. Serve and enjoy.

Nutrition:
Calories 81 Fat 4 g Carbohydrates 10.7 g
Sugar 2.5 g Protein 4 g
Cholesterol 0 mg

Baked Artichoke Hearts

Preparation Time: 10 minutes
Cooking Time: 25 minutes
Servings: 6
Ingredients:

- 18 oz frozen artichoke hearts, defrosted
- 1 tablespoon olive oil

- Pepper
- Salt

Directions:

1. Brush artichoke hearts with oil and season with pepper and salt.
2. Select Bake mode.
3. Set time to 25 minutes and temperature 400 F then press START.
4. The air fryer display will prompt you to ADD FOOD once the temperature is reached then place artichoke hearts in the air fryer basket.
5. Serve and enjoy.

Nutrition:
Calories 60
Fat 2.5 g
Carbohydrates 9 g
Sugar 0.8 g
Protein 2.8 g
Cholesterol 0 mg

Mushrooms Cauliflower Roast

Preparation Time: 10 minutes
Cooking Time: 25 minutes
Servings: 6
Ingredients:

- 1 lb mushrooms, cleaned
- 10 garlic cloves, peeled
- 2 cups cauliflower florets
- 1 tablespoon fresh parsley, chopped
- 1 tablespoon Italian seasoning
- 2 tablespoon olive oil
- Pepper
- Salt

Directions:

1. Add cauliflower, mushrooms, Italian seasoning, olive oil, garlic, pepper, and salt into the mixing bowl and toss well.
2. Transfer cauliflower and mushroom mixture in baking dish.
3. Select Bake mode.
4. Set time to 25 minutes and temperature 400 F then press START.
5. The air fryer display will prompt you to ADD FOOD once the temperature is reached then place the baking dish in the air fryer basket.
6. Serve and enjoy.

Nutrition:
Calories 90 Fat 5.8 g Carbohydrates 8.5 g
Sugar 3.9 g
Protein 3.9 g
Cholesterol 0 mg

Snacks

Cheddar Artichoke Dip

Preparation time: 15 minutes
Cooking time: 27 minutes
Servings: 7
Ingredients:

- 1 cup spinach
- 8 oz. artichoke, chopped
- ½ cup heavy cream
- 5 oz. Cheddar cheese
- ¼ teaspoon salt
- 1 teaspoon paprika
- ½ teaspoon ground coriander
- ½ cup cream cheese

- ½ teaspoon garlic powder
- 1 teaspoon olive oil

Directions:

1. Put the chopped artichoke in foil.
2. Sprinkle with the salt, paprika, garlic powder, and ground coriander.
3. Drizzle the artichokes with olive oil.
4. Wrap the artichoke in foil.
5. Preheat the air fryer to 360 F.
6. Place the wrapped artichoke in the air fryer and cook it for 25 minutes.
7. Meanwhile, chop the spinach roughly and place it in a blender.
8. Add the heavy cream, salt, paprika, ground coriander, and cream cheese.
9. Blend until well combined.
10. Remove the artichoke from the air fryer and add to the spinach mixture.
11. Blend for 2 minutes.
12. Pour the blended mixture into the air fryer.
13. Add heavy cream.
14. Shred Cheddar cheese and add it to the air fryer.
15. Stir and cook for 3 minutes at 360 F.
16. When the cheese is melted – the dip is cooked.
17. Serve warm.

Nutrition:
calories 192,
fat 16.4,
fiber 2,
carbs 4.8,
protein 7.7

Delicious Broccoli Tots

Preparation Time: 10 minutes

Cooking Time: 16 minutes

Serve: 4

Ingredients:

- 1 egg
- 2 tbsp almond flour
- 2 cups cheddar cheese, shredded
- 2 cups cauliflower rice, cooked
- 1 tsp Italian seasoning
- Pepper
- Salt

Directions:

1. Add all ingredients into the mixing bowl and mix until well combined.
2. Make small balls from mixture and place on a cooking tray.
3. Place drip pan into the bottom of the vortex plus air fryer oven cooking chamber.
4. Select BAKE mode, then set the temperature to 400 F and the time to 16 minutes, then press start.
5. When the display shows Add Food then place the cooking tray in the vortex plus air fryer oven.

6. Turn broccoli tots halfway through.

7. Serve and enjoy.

Nutrition:

Calories 322

Fat 24.4 g

Carbohydrates 8.2 g

Sugar 1.1 g

Protein 17.7 g

Cholesterol 101 mg

Cinnamon Pumpkin Fries
Preparation time: 15 minutes
Cooking time: 15 minutes
Servings: 7
Ingredients:
- 1-pound pumpkin
- 1 teaspoon ground cinnamon
- ½ teaspoon ground ginger
- ½ teaspoon salt
- 1 teaspoon olive oil
- 1 teaspoon turmeric

Directions:
1. Peel the pumpkin and cut it into thick strips.
2. Coat the pumpkin strips with the ground cinnamon, ground ginger, salt, and turmeric.
3. Stir the pumpkin carefully and leave for 5 minutes to marinade.
4. Preheat the air fryer to 360 F.
5. Drizzle the pumpkin with the olive oil and transfer it to the air fryer basket.
6. Cook the pumpkin fries for 15 minutes, stirring occasionally.
7. Place the cooked pumpkin fries on paper towel.
8. Chill them for 3-4 minutes before serving.

Nutrition:
calories 30, fat 0.9, fiber 2.2, carbs 5.8, protein 0.8

Winter Squash & Pumpkin Tots
Preparation time: 15 minutes
Cooking time: 10 minutes
Servings: 7
Ingredients:
- 1 cup pumpkin puree
- 1 tablespoon almond flour
- ½ teaspoon ground nutmeg
- ¼ teaspoon salt
- ¼ cup coconut flour
- 1 teaspoon olive oil
- ¼ teaspoon turmeric

Directions:
1. Take a large bowl and combine the pumpkin puree, almond flour, ground nutmeg, salt, and turmeric.
2. Mix using a fork.
3. Add coconut flour.
4. Mix again. The pumpkin mixture should be non-sticky.
5. Separate the pumpkin dough into 5 and form 5 tots.
6. Preheat the air fryer to 360 F.

7. Grease the air fryer with the olive oil and cook the pumpkin tots for 10 minutes.

Nutrition:

calories 62, fat 3.6,
fiber 3.5, carbs 7.3, protein 1.9

Bacon Shrimps

Preparation time: 10 minutes
Cooking time: 10 minutes
Servings: 4
Ingredients:

- 8 oz.shrimp
- 5 oz. bacon, sliced
- 1 teaspoon fresh lemon juice
- ¼ teaspoon salt
- ¼ teaspoon turmeric
- ½ tablespoon olive oil
- ½ teaspoon dried rosemary

Directions:

1. Peel the shrimps and coat them with fresh lemon juice and salt.
2. Mix using your hands.
3. Sprinkle the shrimp with turmeric and dried rosemary.
4. Wrap the shrimp in sliced bacon.
5. Secure with toothpicks.
6. Preheat the air fryer to 360 F.
7. Grease the air fryer with olive oil.
8. Put the shrimps in the air fryer and cook them for 5 minutes on each side.

Nutrition:

calories 276,
fat 17.6,
fiber 0.1,
carbs 1.6,

protein 26.1

Dessert

Soft Turmeric Cookies

Preparation Time: 10 minutes
Cooking time: 20 minutes
Servings: 12
Ingredients:

- 2 eggs, beaten
- 1 tablespoon coconut cream
- 3 tablespoons coconut oil, melted
- 2 teaspoons ground turmeric
- 1 teaspoon vanilla extract
- 2.5 cup coconut flour
- 2 tablespoons Erythritol

Directions:

1. Mix all ingredients in the mixing bowl.
2. Knead the dough and make the cookies using the cutter.
3. Put the cookies in the air fryer basket and cook at 350F for 20 minutes.

Nutrition:

calories 147,
fat 17,
fiber 10.1,
carbs 17.6,
protein 4.3

Vanilla Scones

Preparation time: 20 minutes
Cooking time: 10 minutes
Servings: 6
Ingredients:

- 4 oz coconut flour

- ½ teaspoon baking powder
- 1 teaspoon apple cider vinegar
- 2 teaspoons mascarpone
- ¼ cup heavy cream
- 1 teaspoon vanilla extract
- 1 tablespoon Erythritol
- Cooking spray

Directions:

1. In the mixing bowl, mix coconut flour with baking powder, apple cider vinegar, mascarpone, heavy cream, vanilla extract, and Erythritol.
2. Knead the dough and cut into scones.
3. Then put them in the air fryer basket and sprinkle with cooking spray.
4. Cook the vanilla scones at 365F for 10 minutes.

Nutrition:
calories 104,
fat 4.1,
fiber 8.1,
carbs 14,
protein 3

Mint Pie

Preparation time: 15 minutes
Cooking time: 25 minutes
Servings: 2
Ingredients:

- 1 tablespoon instant coffee
- 2 tablespoons almond butter, softened
- 2 tablespoons Erythritol
- 1 teaspoon dried mint
- 3 eggs, beaten
- 1 teaspoon spearmint, dried
- 4 teaspoons coconut flour
- Cooking spray

Directions:

1. Spray the air fryer basket with cooking spray.
2. Then mix all ingredients in the mixer bowl.
3. When you get a smooth mixture, transfer it in the air fryer basket. Flatten it gently.
4. Cook the pie at 365F for 25 minutes.

Nutrition:
calories 313,
fat 19.6,
fiber 11.7,
carbs 19.6,
protein 15.7

Saffron Cookies

Preparation Time: 10 minutes
Cooking time: 15 minutes
Servings: 12
Ingredients:

- 2 cups coconut flour
- ½ cup Erythritol
- ¼ cup coconut, melted
- 1 egg, beaten
- 2 teaspoons saffron
- 1 teaspoon vanilla extract

Directions:

1. Mix all ingredients in the bowl and knead the dough.
2. Make the cookies and put them in the air fryer basket in one layer.
3. Cook the cookies at 355F for 15 minutes.

Nutrition:
calories 106,
fat 4.3,
fiber 8.2,
carbs 12.4,
protein 4.5

CHAPTER 8:

June

Lunch

Lettuce Salad with Beef Strips

Preparation time: 10 minutes
Cooking time: 12 minutes
Servings: 5
Ingredients:

- 2 cup lettuce
- 10 oz. beef brisket
- 2 tablespoon sesame oil
- 1 tablespoon sunflower seeds
- 1 cucumber
- 1 teaspoon ground black pepper
- 1 teaspoon paprika
- 1 teaspoon Italian spices
- 2 teaspoon butter
- 1 teaspoon dried dill
- 2 tablespoon coconut milk

Directions:

1. Cut the beef brisket into strips.
2. Sprinkle the beef strips with the ground black pepper, paprika, and dried dill.
3. Preheat the air fryer to 365 F.
4. Put the butter in the air fryer basket tray and melt it.
5. Then add the beef strips and cook them for 6 minutes on each side.
6. Meanwhile, tear the lettuce and toss it in a big salad bowl.
7. Crush the sunflower seeds and sprinkle over the lettuce.
8. Chop the cucumber into the small cubes and add to the salad bowl.
9. Then combine the sesame oil and Italian spices together. Stir the oil..
10. Combine the lettuce mixture with the coconut milk and stir it using 2 wooden spatulas.
11. When the meat is cooked – let it chill to room temperature.
12. Add the beef strips to the salad bowl.
13. Stir it gently and sprinkle the salad with the sesame oil dressing.
14. Serve the dish immediately.

Nutrition:
calories 199,
fat 12.4,
fiber 0.9,
carbs 3.9,
protein 18.1

Cayenne Rib Eye Steak

Preparation time: 10 minutes
Cooking time: 13 minutes
Servings: 2
Ingredients:

- 1-pound rib eye steak
- 1 teaspoon salt
- 1 teaspoon cayenne pepper
- ½ teaspoon chili flakes
- 3 tablespoon cream
- 1 teaspoon olive oil
- 1 teaspoon lemongrass
- 1 tablespoon butter
- 1 teaspoon garlic powder

Directions:

1. Preheat the air fryer to 360 F.
2. Take a shallow bowl and combine the cayenne pepper, salt, chili flakes, lemongrass, and garlic powder together.
3. Mix the spices gently.
4. Sprinkle the rib eye steak with the spice mixture.
5. Melt the butter and combine it with cream and olive oil.
6. Churn the mixture.
7. Pour the churned mixture into the air fryer basket tray.
8. Add the rib eye steak.
9. Cook the steak for 13 minutes. Do not stir the steak during the cooking.
10. When the steak is cooked transfer it to a paper towel to soak all the excess fat.
11. Serve the steak. You can slice the steak if desired.

Nutrition:
calories 708,
fat 59,
fiber 0.4,
carbs 2.3,
protein 40.4

Beef-Chicken Meatball Casserole

Preparation time: 15 minutes
Cooking time: 21 minutes
Servings: 7
Ingredients:

- 1 eggplants
- 10 oz. ground chicken
- 8 oz. ground beef
- 1 teaspoon minced garlic
- 1 teaspoon ground white pepper
- 1 egg
- 1 tablespoon coconut flour
- 8 oz. Parmesan, shredded
- 2 tablespoon butter
- 1/3 cup cream

Directions:

1. Combine the ground chicken and ground beef in a large bowl.
2. Add the minced garlic and ground white pepper.
3. Crack the egg into the bowl with the ground meat mixture and stir it carefully until well combined.
4. Then add the coconut flour and mix.
5. Make small meatballs from the ground meat.
6. Preheat the air fryer to 360 F.

7. Sprinkle the air fryer basket tray with the butter and pour the cream.
8. Peel the eggplant and chop it.
9. Put the meatballs over the cream and sprinkle them with the chopped eggplant.
10. Make a layer of shredded cheese.
11. Put the casserole in the air fryer and cook it for 21 minutes.
12. Let the casserole cool to room temperature before serving.

Nutrition:
calories 314,
fat 16.8,
fiber 3.4,
carbs 7.5,
protein 33.9

Juicy Pork Chops
Preparation time: 10 minutes
Cooking time: 11 minutes
Servings: 3
Ingredients:
- 1 teaspoon peppercorns
- 1 teaspoon kosher salt
- 1 teaspoon minced garlic
- ½ teaspoon dried rosemary
- 1 tablespoon butter
- 13 oz. pork chops

Directions:
1. Rub the pork chops with the dried rosemary, minced garlic, and kosher salt.
2. Preheat the air fryer to 365 F.
3. Put the butter and peppercorns in the air fryer basket tray. Melt the butter.
4. Place the pork chops in the melted butter.
5. Cook the pork chops for 6 minutes.
6. Turn the pork chops over.
7. Cook the pork chops for 5 minutes more.
8. When the meat is cooked dry gently with a paper towel.
9. Serve the juicy pork chops immediately.

Nutrition:
calories 431,
fat 34.4,
fiber 0.3,
carbs 0.9,
protein 27.8

Chicken Goulash
Preparation time: 10 minutes
Cooking time: 17 minutes
Servings: 6
Ingredients:
- 4 oz chive stems
- 2 green peppers, chopped
- 1 teaspoon olive oil
- 14 oz. ground chicken
- ½ cup chicken stock
- 2 garlic cloves, sliced
- 1 teaspoon salt
- 1 teaspoon ground black pepper
- 1 teaspoon mustard

Directions:

1. Chop chives roughly.
2. Spray the air fryer basket tray with the olive oil.
3. Preheat the air fryer to 365 F.
4. Put the chopped chives in the air fryer basket tray.
5. Add the chopped green pepper and cook the vegetables for 5 minutes.
6. Add the ground chicken.
7. Cook the mixture for 6 minutes more.
8. Add the chicken stock, sliced garlic cloves, salt, ground black pepper, and mustard.
9. Mix well to combine.
10. Cook the goulash for 6 minutes more.

Nutrition:
calories 161,
fat 6.1,
fiber 1.7,
carbs 6,
protein 20.3

<u>Dinner</u>

Basil-Garlic Breaded Chicken Bake

Intermediate Recipe
Preparation Time: 5 minutes
Cooking Time: 30 minutes
Serving: 2
Ingredients:

- 2 boneless skinless chicken breast halves (4 ounces each)
- 1 tablespoon butter, melted
- 2 garlic cloves, minced
- 1 1/2 tablespoons minced fresh basil
- 1/2 tablespoon olive oil
- 1/2 teaspoon salt
- 1/4 cup all-purpose flour
- 1/4 cup egg substitute
- 1/4 cup grated Parmesan cheese
- 1/4 cup dry bread crumbs
- 1/4 teaspoon pepper

Directions:

1. In shallow bowl, whisk well egg substitute and place flour in a separate bowl. Dip chicken in flour, then egg, and then flour. In a small bowl whisk well the butter, bread crumbs and cheese. Sprinkle over chicken.
2. Lightly grease baking pan of air fryer with cooking spray. Place breaded chicken on bottom of pan. Cover with foil.
3. For 20 minutes, cook it on 390 F.
4. Meanwhile, in a bowl whisk well remaining ingredient.
5. Remove foil from pan and then pour over chicken the remaining Ingredients. Cook for 8 minutes. Serve and enjoy.

Nutrition:
Calories 311
Carbs 22.0g
Protein 31.0g
Fat 11.0g

BBQ Chicken Recipe from Greece

Basic Recipe
Preparation Time: 5 minutes
Cooking Time: 24minutes
Serving: 2
Ingredients:

- 1 (8 ounce) container fat-free plain yogurt
- 2 tablespoons fresh lemon juice
- 2 teaspoons dried oregano
- 1-pound skinless, boneless chicken breast halves - cut into 1-inch pieces
- 1 large red onion, cut into wedges
- 1/2 teaspoon lemon zest
- 1/2 teaspoon salt
- 1 large green bell pepper, cut into 1 1/2-inch pieces
- 1/4 teaspoon ground black pepper
- 1/4 teaspoon crushed dried rosemary

Directions:

1. In a shallow dish, mix well rosemary, pepper, salt, oregano, lemon juice, lemon zest, feta cheese, and yogurt. Add chicken and toss well to coat. Marinate in the ref for 3 hours.
2. Thread bell pepper, onion, and chicken pieces in skewers. Place on skewer rack.
3. For 12 minutes, cook it on 360oF. Turnover skewershalfway through cooking time. If needed, cook in batches.
4. Serve and enjoy.

Nutrition:
Calories 242

Carbs 12.3g
Protein 31.0g
Fat 7.5g

BBQ Teriyaki Glazed Chicken

Basic Recipe
Preparation Time: 5 minutes
Cooking Time: 20 minutes
Serving: 2
Ingredients:

- ¼ teaspoon pepper
- ½ cup brown sugar
- ½ cup soy sauce
- ½ teaspoon salt
- 1 green bell pepper, cut into 1-inch cubes
- 1 red bell pepper, cut into 1-inch cubes
- 1 red onion, cut into 1-inch cubes
- 1 Tablespoon glucomannan
- 1 Tablespoon water
- 1 yellow red bell pepper, cut into 1-inch cubes
- 2 boneless skinless chicken breasts cut into 1-inch cubes
- 2 garlic cloves, minced
- Green onions, for garnish

Directions:

1. In a saucepan, bring to a boil salt, pepper, garlic, soy sauce, and brown sugar. In a small bowl whisk well, glucomannan and water. Slowly stir in to mixture in pan while whisking constantly. Simmer until thickened, around 3 minutes. Save ¼ cup of the sauce for basting and set aside.
2. In shallow dish, mix well chicken and remaining thickened sauce.

Toss well to coat. Marinate in the ref for a half hour.

3. Thread bell pepper, onion, and chicken pieces in skewers. Place on skewer rack in air fryer.
4. For 10 minutes, cook on 360oF. Turnover skewers halfway through cooking time. and baste with sauce. If needed, cook in batches.
5. Serve and enjoy with a sprinkle of green onions.

Nutrition:
Calories 391
Carbs 58.7g
Protein 31.2g
Fat 3.4g

BBQ Turkey Meatballs with Cranberry Sauce
Basic Recipe
Preparation Time: 5 minutes
Cooking Time: 20 minutes
Serving: 4
Ingredients:

- 1 ½ tablespoons of water
- 2 teaspoons cider vinegar
- 1 tsp. salt and more to taste
- 1-pound ground turkey
- 1 1/2 tablespoons barbecue sauce
- 1/3 cup cranberry sauce
- 1/4-pound ground bacon

Directions:

1. In a bowl, mix well with hands the turkey, ground bacon and a tsp. of salt. Evenly form into 16 equal sized balls.

2. In a small saucepan boil cranberry sauce, barbecue sauce, water, cider vinegar, and a dash or two of salt. Mix well and simmer for 3 minutes
3. Thread meatballs in skewers and baste with cranberry sauce. Place on skewer rack in air fryer.
4. For 15 minutes, cook it on 360oF. Every after 5 minutes of cooking time, turnover skewers and baste with sauce. If needed, cook in batches.
5. Serve and enjoy.

Nutrition:
Calories 217 Carbs 11.5g
Protein 28.0g
Fat 10.9g

Blueberry Overload French Toast
Basic Recipe
Preparation Time: 5 minutes
Cooking Time: 40minutes
Serving: 5
Ingredients:

- 1 (8 ounce) package cream cheese, cut into 1-inch cubes
- 1 cup fresh blueberries, divided
- 1 cup milk
- 1 tablespoon glucomannan
- 1/2 cup water
- 1/2 cup white sugar
- 1/2 teaspoon vanilla extract
- 1-1/2 teaspoons butter
- 2 tablespoons and 2 teaspoons maple syrup
- 6 eggs, beaten
- 6 slices day-old bread, cut into 1-inch cubes

Directions:

1. Lightly grease baking pan of air fryer with cooking spray.
2. Evenly spread half of the bread on bottom of pan. Sprinkle evenly the cream cheese and ½ cup blueberries. Add remaining bread on top.
3. In a large bowl, whisk well eggs, milk, syrup, and vanilla extract. Pour over bread mixture.
4. Cover air fryer baking pan with foil and refrigerate overnight.
5. Preheat air fryer to 330oF.
6. Cook for 25 minutes covered in foil, remove foil and cook for another 20 minutes or until middle is set. Meanwhile, make the sauce by mixing glucomannan, water, and sugar in a saucepan and bring to a boil. Stir in remaining blueberries and simmer until thickened and blueberries have burst.
7. Serve and enjoy with blueberry syrup.

Nutrition:
Calories 492 Carbs 51.9g Protein 15.1g
 Fat 24.8g

Cauliflower Rice 'n Cheese Casserole

Basic Recipe
Preparation Time: 5 minutes
Cooking Time: 30 minutes
Serving: 4
Ingredients:

- 1 (10 ounce) can chunk chicken, Dry out
- 1 cup cooked cauliflower rice
- 1 cup water
- 1/2 (10.75 ounce) can condensed cream of chicken soup
- 1/2 (10.75 ounce) can condensed cream of mushroom soup
- 1/2 cup milk
- 1/2 small white onion, chopped
- 1/2-pound processed cheese food
- 2 tablespoons butter
- 8-ounce frozen chopped broccoli

Directions:

1. Lightly grease baking pan of air fryer with cooking spray. Add water and bring to a boil at 390oF. Stir in cauliflower rice and cook for 3 minutes.
2. Stir in processed cheese, onion, broccoli, milk, butter, chicken soup, mushroom soup, and chicken. Mix well. Cook for 15 minutes at 390oF, fluff mixture and continue cooking for another 10 minutes until tops are browned. Serve and enjoy.

Nutrition:
Calories 752 Carbs 82.7g
Protein 36.0g Fat 30.8g

Meat

Flavorful Burger Patties

Preparation Time: 10 minutes
Cooking Time: 15 minutes
Servings: 4
Ingredients:

- 1 lb ground lamb
- 1/4 teaspoon cayenne pepper
- 1/4 cup fresh parsley, chopped
- 1/4 cup onion, minced

- 1 tablespoon garlic, minced
- 1/2 teaspoon ground allspice
- 1 teaspoon ground cinnamon
- 1 teaspoon ground coriander
- 1 teaspoon ground cumin
- 1/4 teaspoon pepper
- 1 teaspoon kosher salt

Directions:

1. Add all ingredients into the large bowl and mix until well combined.
2. Make 4 patties from the meat mixture.
3. Select Bake mode.
4. Set time to 14 minutes and temperature 375 F then press START.
5. The air fryer display will prompt you to ADD FOOD once the temperature is reached then place patties in the air fryer basket. Turn patties halfway through.
6. Serve and enjoy.

Nutrition:
Calories 223
Fat 8.5 g
Carbohydrates 2.6 g
Sugar 0.4 g
Protein 32.3 g
Cholesterol 102 mg

Meatballs

Preparation Time: 10 minutes
Cooking Time: 20 minutes
Servings: 4
Ingredients:

- 1 lb ground lamb
- 2 tablespoon fresh parsley, chopped
- 1 tablespoon garlic, minced
- 1 egg, lightly beaten
- 1/4 teaspoon red pepper flakes
- 1 teaspoon ground cumin
- 2 teaspoon fresh oregano, chopped
- 1/4 teaspoon pepper
- 1 teaspoon kosher salt

Directions:

1. Add all ingredients into the mixing bowl and mix until well combined.
2. Make small meatballs from meat mixture.
3. Select Bake mode.
4. Set time to 20 minutes and temperature 400 F then press START.
5. The air fryer display will prompt you to ADD FOOD once the temperature is reached then place meatballs in the air fryer basket.
6. Serve and enjoy.

Nutrition:
Calories 235
Fat 9.7 g
Carbohydrates 1.7 g
Sugar 0.2 g
Protein 33.6 g
Cholesterol 143 mg

Pork And Mixed Greens Salad

Preparation Time: 10 minutes
Cooking Time: 15 minutes
Servings: 4
Ingredients:

- 2 pounds pork tenderloin, cut into 1-inch slices (see Tip)
- 1 teaspoon olive oil
- 1 teaspoon dried marjoram
- $\frac{1}{8}$ teaspoon freshly ground black pepper
- 6 cups mixed salad greens

- 1 red bell pepper, sliced (see Tip)
- 1 (8-ounce) package button mushrooms, sliced (see Tip)
- ⅓ cup low-sodium low-fat vinaigrette dressing

Directions:
1. In a medium bowl, mix the pork slices and olive oil. Toss to coat.
2. Sprinkle with the marjoram and pepper and rub these into the pork.
3. Grill the pork in the air fryer, in batches, for about 4 to 6 minutes, or until the pork reaches at least 145°F on a meat thermometer.
4. Meanwhile, in a serving bowl, mix the salad greens, red bell pepper, and mushrooms. Toss gently.
5. When the pork is cooked, add the slices to the salad. -Drizzle with the vinaigrette and toss gently. Serve immediately.

Nutrition:
Calories: 172
Fat: 5 g
Saturated Fat: 1g
Protein: 27g
Carbohydrates: 28g
Sodium: 124mg
Fiber: 2g
Sugar: 3g

Fish

Baked Salmon Patties
Preparation Time: 10 minutes
Cooking Time: 20 minutes
Servings: 4
Ingredients:

- 2 eggs, lightly beaten
- 12 oz can salmon, skinless, boneless, and drained
- 1/2 cup almond flour
- 1/2 teaspoon pepper
- 1 tablespoon Dijon mustard
- 1 teaspoon garlic powder
- 2 tablespoon fresh parsley, chopped
- 1/2 cup celery, diced
- 1/2 cup bell pepper, diced
- 1/2 cup onion, diced

Directions:
1. Add salmon and remaining ingredients into the mixing bowl and mix until well combined.
2. Make 8 equal shapes of patties from the mixture.
3. Place the cooking tray in the air fryer basket. Line air fryer basket with parchment paper.
4. Select Bake mode.
5. Set time to 20 minutes and temperature 400 F then press START.
6. The air fryer display will prompt you to ADD FOOD once the temperature is reached then place patties in the air fryer basket.
7. Turn patties halfway through.
8. Serve and enjoy.

Nutrition:
Calories 182 Fat 6.5 g
Carbohydrates 4.8 g
Sugar 2.1 g Protein 22.9 g
Cholesterol 105 mg

Healthy Swordfish Fillets

Preparation Time: 10 minutes
Cooking Time: 20 minutes
Servings: 2
Ingredients:

- 12 oz swordfish fillets
- 1 garlic clove, minced
- 2 teaspoon fresh parsley, chopped
- 3 tablespoon olive oil
- 1/2 teaspoon lemon zest, grated
- 1/2 teaspoon ginger, grated
- 1/8 teaspoon crushed red pepper

Directions:

1. In a small bowl, mix together 2 tablespoon oil, lemon zest, red pepper, ginger, garlic, and parsley.
2. Season fish fillets with salt.
3. Heat remaining oil in a pan over medium-high heat.
4. Place fish fillets in the pan and cook until lightly browned 2-3 minutes.
5. Select Bake mode.
6. Set time to 10 minutes and temperature 400 F then press START.
7. The air fryer display will prompt you to ADD FOOD once the temperature is reached then place fish fillets in the air fryer basket.
8. Pour oil mixture over fish fillets and serve.

Nutrition:
Calories 449 Fat 29.8 g
Carbohydrates 1.1 g Sugar 0.1 g
Protein 43.4 g Cholesterol 85 mg

Vegetable

Lemon Garlic Cauliflower

Preparation Time: 10 minutes
Cooking Time: 35 minutes
Servings: 4
Ingredients:

- 6 cups cauliflower florets
- 5 garlic cloves, chopped
- 1/4 fresh lemon juice
- 2 tablespoon olive oil
- 1/2 teaspoon onion powder
- 1/4 teaspoon cayenne
- Pepper
- Salt

Directions:

1. Add all ingredients into the large bowl and toss well.
2. Select Roast mode.
3. Set time to 35 minutes and temperature 400 F then press START.
4. The air fryer display will prompt you to ADD FOOD once the temperature is reached then add cauliflower florets in the air fryer basket. Stir halfway through.
5. Serve and enjoy.

Nutrition:
Calories 105
Fat 7.2 g
Carbohydrates 9.6 g
Sugar 3.8 g
Protein 3.3 g
Cholesterol 0 mg

Eggplant Zucchini Casserole

Preparation Time: 10 minutes

Cooking Time: 35 minutes

Serve: 6

Ingredients:

- 3 zucchinis, sliced
- 1 medium eggplant, sliced
- 1 tbsp olive oil
- 3 garlic cloves, minced
- 4 tbsp basil, chopped
- 3 oz parmesan cheese, grated
- 1/4 cup parsley, chopped
- 1/4 tsp pepper
- 1/4 tsp salt

Directions:

1. Add all ingredients into the large bowl and toss well to combine.
2. Pour eggplant mixture into a greased baking dish.
3. Select BAKE mode, then set the temperature to 350 F and the time to 35 minutes, then press start.
4. When the display shows Add Food then place the baking dish in the vortex plus air fryer oven.
5. Serve and enjoy.

Nutrition:

Calories 109

Fat 5.8 g

Carbohydrates 10.2 g

Sugar 4.8 g

Protein 7 g

Cholesterol 10 mg

Delicious Ratatouille

Preparation Time: 10 minutes
Cooking Time: 15 minutes
Servings: 6
Ingredients:

- 1 eggplant, diced
- 1 tablespoon vinegar
- 1 onion, diced
- 2 bell peppers, diced
- 1 1/2 tablespoon olive oil
- 2 tablespoon herb de Provence
- 3 garlic cloves, chopped
- Pepper
- Salt

Directions:

1. Add all ingredients into the bowl and toss well and transfer into the baking dish.
2. Select Air Fry mode.
3. Set time to 15 minutes and temperature 400 F then press START.
4. The air fryer display will prompt you to ADD FOOD once the temperature is reached then place the baking

dish in the air fryer basket. Stir halfway through.

5. Serve and enjoy.

Nutrition:
Calories 72
Fat 4 g
Carbohydrates 8.5 g
Sugar 4.9 g
Protein 2 g
Cholesterol 0 mg

Snacks

Avocado in Bacon Wraps

Preparation time: 15 minutes
Cooking time: 11 minutes
Servings: 8
Ingredients:

- 2 avocado, pitted
- 1 egg
- 1 tablespoon coconut flakes
- ½ teaspoon salt
- 1 teaspoon paprika
- 1 teaspoon turmeric
- ½ teaspoon ground black pepper
- 1 teaspoon olive oil
- 5 oz. bacon, sliced
- 1 teaspoon dried rosemary

Directions:

1. Peel the avocados and cut them into medium strips.

2. Crack the egg in a bowl and whisk it.

3. Sprinkle the whisked egg with the coconut flakes, salt, paprika, turmeric, ground black pepper, and dried rosemary.

4. Put the avocado strips in the egg mixture.

5. Then wrap the avocado in the sliced bacon.

6. Preheat the air fryer to 360 F.

7. Place the wrapped avocado sticks in the air fryer rack.

8. Cook for 6 minutes on one side.

9. Turn the avocado over.

10. Cook for 5 minutes more and serve.

Nutrition:
calories 216,
fat 18.6,
fiber 3.7,
carbs 5.2,
protein 8.3

Herbed Crab Cakes

Preparation time: 15 minutes
Cooking time: 10 minutes
Servings: 6
Ingredients:

- 12 oz crabmeat
- ¼ teaspoon salt
- 1 teaspoon chili powder
- 1 teaspoon ground white pepper
- 1 egg
- 1 tablespoon almond flour
- 1 tablespoon butter
- 1 tablespoon chives

Directions:

1. Chop the crabmeat into small pieces and place in a bowl.

2. Sprinkle the crabmeat with salt, chili powder, ground white pepper, and chives.

3. Stir the mixture gently with a spoon.

4. Then crack the egg into the crabmeat.

5. Add almond flour and stir carefully until you have a smooth texture.

6. Preheat the air fryer to 400 F.

7. Take 2 spoons and place a small amount of the crabmeat mixture in one of them.

8. Cover it with the second spoon and make the crab cake.

9. Toss the butter in the air fryer and melt it.

10. Transfer the crab cakes to the air fryer and cook them for 10 minutes turning halfway through.

11. Cool before serving.

Nutrition:
calories 107,
fat 6.1,
fiber 0.8,
carbs 2.6,
protein 9.1

Jalapeno Bacon Bites

Preparation time: 15 minutes
Cooking time: 11 minutes
Servings: 5
Ingredients:

- 6 oz. bacon, sliced
- 1 cup jalapeno pepper
- ½ teaspoon salt
- ½ teaspoon paprika
- 1 teaspoon olive oil

Directions:

1. Wash the jalapeno peppers carefully.

2. Combine the salt, paprika, and olive oil together.

3. Stir gently.

4. Brush the jalapeno peppers with the olive oil mixture generously.

5. Wrap each jalapeno pepper in the bacon slices.

6. Secure the jalapeno bites with toothpicks.

7. Preheat the air fryer to 360 F.

8. Put the jalapeno bites in the air fryer rack.

9. Cook for 11 minutes or until the bacon is crisp.

10. Transfer the cooked jalapeno pepper bites to a plate and cover them with paper towels to remove excess grease before serving.

Nutrition:
calories 198,
fat 15.3,
fiber 0.6,
carbs 1.7,
protein 12.9

Chicken Nuggets

Preparation time: 15 minutes
Cooking time: 10 minutes
Servings: 7
Ingredients:

- 1-pound chicken fillet
- ½ teaspoon salt
- ½ teaspoon ground black pepper
- ½ teaspoon chili pepper
- 2 egg
- ½ cup coconut flour

Directions:

1. Cut the chicken fillet into nugget size pieces.

2. Crack the eggs into a bowl and whisk them.

3. Combine the coconut flour, chili pepper, salt, and ground black pepper in a large mixing bowl.

4. Mix well to combine.

5. Dip the nuggets in the whisked egg.

6. Coat the chicken nuggets in the almond flour mixture.

7. Preheat the air fryer to 360 F.

8. Transfer the coated chicken nuggets to the air fryer rack and cook for 10 minutes.

9. Serve hot.

Nutrition:
calories 212,
fat 7.4,
fiber 3.9,
carbs 6.8,
protein 23.1

Dessert

Keto Balls
Preparation time: 15 minutes
Cooking time: 4 minutes
Servings: 10
Ingredients:

- 2 eggs, beaten
- 1 teaspoon coconut oil, melted
- 9 oz coconut flour
- 5 oz provolone cheese, shredded
- 2 tablespoons Erythritol
- 1 teaspoon baking powder
- ¼ teaspoon ground coriander
- Cooking spray

Directions:

1. Mix eggs with coconut oil, coconut flour, Provolone cheese, Erythritol, baking powder, and ground cinnamon.

2. Make the balls and put them in the air fryer basket.

3. Sprinkle the balls with cooking spray and cook at 400F for 4 minutes.

Nutrition:
calories 176,
fat 7.8,
fiber 10.9,
carbs 18.9,
protein 8.4

Sage Muffins
Preparation Time: 10 minutes
Cooking time: 20 minutes
Servings: 8
Ingredients:

- 3 tablespoons coconut oil, softened
- 1 egg, beaten
- ½ cup Erythritol
- ¼ cup almond flour
- 1 teaspoon dried sage
- 3 tablespoons mascarpone
- ½ teaspoon baking soda
- Cooking spray

Directions:

1. Spray the muffin molds with cooking spray.

2. Then mix all ingredients in the mixing bowl and stir until smooth.

3. Pour the mixture in the muffin molds and transfer in the air fryer.

4. Cook the muffins at 350F for 20 minutes.

Nutrition:
calories 85,
fat 8.3,
fiber 0.4,
carbs 0.9,
protein 1.4

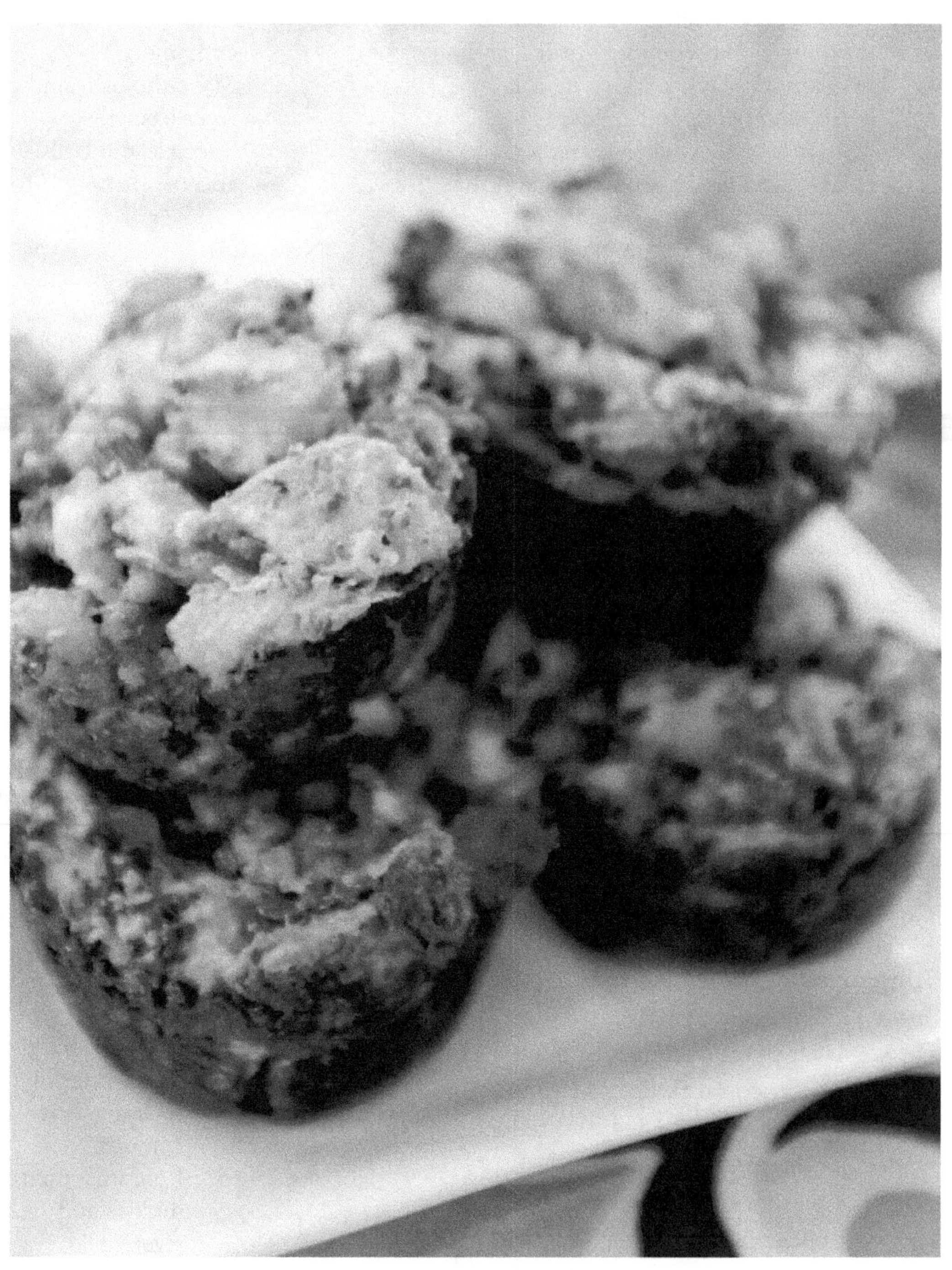

Pecan Tarts

Preparation time: 10 minutes
Cooking time: 10 minutes
Servings: 5
Ingredients:

- 3 pecans, chopped
- ½ cup coconut flour
- 1 egg, beaten
- 1 tablespoon coconut oil, softened
- 1 tablespoon swerve
- ½ teaspoon baking powder
- Cooking spray

Directions:

1. Spray the air fryer basket with cooking spray.
2. Then mix coconut flour with egg, coconut oil, swerve, and baking powder.
3. When you get a smooth batter, pour it in the air fryer basket, flatten gently, and top with pecans.
4. Cook the tart at 375F for 10 minutes.

Nutrition:
calories 143,
fat 10.8,
fiber 5.7,
carbs 9.5,
protein 3.6

Raspberry Jam

Preparation Time: 10 minutes
Cooking time: 20 minutes
Servings: 12
Ingredients:

- ¼ cup Erythritol
- 7 oz raspberries
- 1 tablespoon lime juice
- ¼ cup of water

Directions:

1. Put all ingredients in the air fryer and stir gently.
2. Cook the jam at 350F for 20 minutes. Stir the jam every 5 minutes to avoid burning.

Nutrition:
calories 9,
fat 0.1,
fiber 1.1,
carbs 2,
protein 0.2

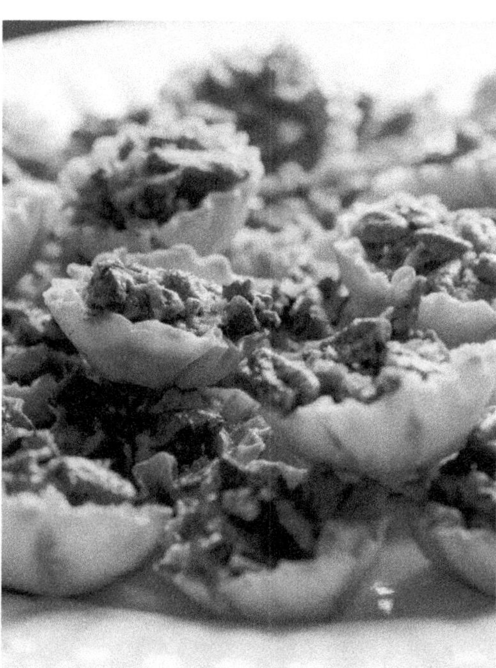

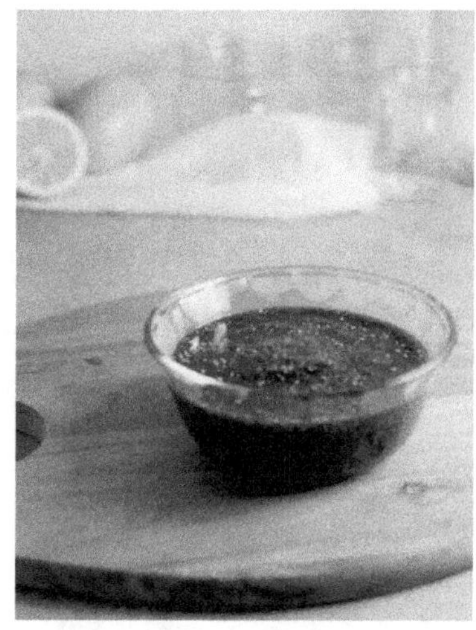

CHAPTER 9:

July

Lunch

Chicken & Turkey Meatloaf
Preparation time: 15 minutes
Cooking time: 25 minutes
Servings: 12
Ingredients:
- 3 tablespoon butter
- 10 oz. ground turkey
- 7 oz. ground chicken
- 1 teaspoon dried dill
- ½ teaspoon ground coriander
- 2 tablespoons almond flour
- 1 tablespoon minced garlic
- 3 oz. fresh spinach
- 1 teaspoon salt
- 1 egg
- ½ tablespoon paprika
- 1 teaspoon sesame oil

Directions:
1. Put the ground turkey and ground chicken in a large bowl.
2. Sprinkle the meat with dried dill, ground coriander, almond flour, minced garlic, salt, and paprika.
3. Then chop the fresh spinach and add it to the ground poultry mixture.
4. Crack the egg into the meat mixture and mix well until you get a smooth texture.
5. Great the air fryer basket tray with the olive oil.
6. Preheat the air fryer to 350 F.
7. Roll the ground meat mixture gently to make the flat layer.
8. Put the butter in the center of the meat layer.
9. Make the shape of the meatloaf from the ground meat mixture. Use your fingertips for this step.
10. Place the Prepared meatloaf in the air fryer basket tray.
11. Cook for 25 minutes.
12. When the meatloaf is cooked allow it to rest before serving.

Nutrition:
calories 142, fat 9.8,
fiber 0.8, carbs 1.7, protein 13

Turkey Meatballs with Dried Dill
Preparation time: 15 minutes
Cooking time: 11 minutes
Servings: 9
Ingredients:
- 1-pound ground turkey
- 1 teaspoon chili flakes

- ¼ cup chicken stock
- 2 tablespoon dried dill
- 1 egg
- 1 teaspoon salt
- 1 teaspoon paprika
- 1 tablespoon coconut flour
- 2 tablespoons heavy cream
- 1 teaspoon olive oil

Directions:

1. Crack the egg in a bowl and whisk it with a fork.
2. Add the ground turkey and chili flakes.
3. Sprinkle the mixture with dried dill, salt, paprika, coconut flour, and mix it up.
4. Make the meatballs from the ground turkey mixture.
5. Preheat the air fryer to 360 F.
6. Grease the air fryer basket tray with the olive oil.
7. Then put the meatballs inside.
8. Cook the meatballs for 6 minutes – for 3 minutes on each side.
9. Sprinkle the meatballs with the heavy cream.
10. Cook the meatballs for 5 minutes more.
11. When the turkey meatballs are cooked – let them rest for 2-3 minutes.

Nutrition:
calories 124,
fat 7.9,
fiber 0.5,
carbs 1.2,
protein 14.8

Parmesan Beef Slices

Preparation time: 14 minutes
Cooking time: 25 minutes
Servings: 4
Ingredients:

- 12 oz. beef brisket
- 1 teaspoon kosher salt
- 7 oz. Parmesan, sliced
- 5 oz chive stems
- 1 teaspoon turmeric
- 1 teaspoon dried oregano
- 2 teaspoon butter

Directions:

1. Slice the beef brisket into 4 slices.
2. Sprinkle every beef slice with the turmeric and dried oregano.
3. Grease the air fryer basket tray with the butter.
4. Put the beef slices inside.
5. Dice the chives.
6. Make a layer using the diced chives over the beef slices.
7. Then make a layer using the Parmesan cheese.
8. Preheat the air fryer to 365 F.
9. Cook the beef slices for 25 minutes.

Nutrition:
calories 348, fat 18, fiber 0.9,
carbs 5, protein 42.1

Chili Beef Jerky

Preparation time: 25 minutes
Cooking time: 2.5 hours
Servings: 6
Ingredients:

- 14 oz. beef flank steak
- 1 teaspoon chili pepper

- 3 tablespoon apple cider vinegar
- 1 teaspoon ground black pepper
- 1 teaspoon onion powder
- 1 teaspoon garlic powder
- ¼ teaspoon liquid smoke

Directions:

1. Slice the beefsteak into the medium strips and then tenderize each piece.
2. Take a bowl and combine the apple cider vinegar, ground black pepper, onion powder, garlic powder, and liquid smoke.
3. Whisk gently with a fork.
4. Then transfer the beef pieces in the Prepared mixture and stir well.
5. Leave the meat to marinade for up to 8 hours.
6. Put the marinated beef pieces in the air fryer rack.
7. Cook the beef jerky for 2.5 hours at 150 F.

Nutrition:
calories 129,
fat 4.1,
fiber 0.2,
carbs 1.1,
protein 20.2

Spinach Beef Heart

Preparation time: 15 minutes
Cooking time: 20 minutes
Servings: 4
Ingredients:

- 1-pound beef heart
- 5 oz chive stems
- ½ cup fresh spinach
- 1 teaspoon salt
- 1 teaspoon ground black pepper
- 3 cups chicken stock
- 1 teaspoon butter

Directions:

1. Remove all the fat from the beef heart.
2. Dice the chives.
3. Chop the fresh spinach.
4. Combine the diced chives, fresh spinach, and butter together. Stir it.
5. Make a cut in the beef heart and fill it with the spinach-chives mixture.
6. Preheat the air fryer to 400 F.
7. Pour the chicken stock into the air fryer basket tray.
8. Sprinkle the Prepared stuffed beef heart with the salt and ground black pepper.
9. Put the beef heart in the air fryer and cook it for 20 minutes.
10. Remove the cooked heart from the air fryer and slice it.
11. Sprinkle the slices with the remaining liquid from the air fryer.

Nutrition:
calories 216,
fat 6.8,
fiber 0.8,
carbs 3.8,
protein 33.3

<u>Dinner</u>

Buffalo Style Chicken Dip
Basic Recipe
Preparation Time: 5 minutes
Cooking Time: 10 minutes
Serving: 4
Ingredients:

- 1 (8 ounce) package cream cheese, softened
- 1 tablespoon shredded pepper Jack cheese
- 1/2 pinch cayenne pepper, for garnish
- 1/2 pinch cayenne pepper, or to taste
- 1/4 cup and 2 tablespoons hot pepper sauce (such as Frank's Reshoot®)
- 1/4 cup blue cheese dressing
- 1/4 cup crumbled blue cheese
- 1/4 cup shredded pepper Jack cheese
- 1/4 teaspoon seafood seasoning (such as Old Bay®)
- 1-1/2 cups diced cooked rotisserie chicken

Directions:

1. Lightly grease baking pan of air fryer with cooking spray. Mix in cayenne pepper, seafood seasoning, crumbled blue cheese, blue cheese dressing, pepper Jack, hot pepper sauce, cream cheese, and chicken.
2. For 15 minutes, cook it on 390 F.
3. Let it stand for 5 minutes and garnish with cayenne pepper.
4. Serve and enjoy.

Nutrition:
Calories 405
Carbs 3.2g
Protein 17.1g
Fat 35.9g

Buttered Spinach-Egg Omelet
Basic Recipe
Preparation Time: 5 minutes
Cooking Time: 10 minutes
Serving: 4
Ingredients:

- ¼ cup coconut milk
- 1 tablespoon melted butter
- 1-pound baby spinach, chopped finely
- 3 tablespoons olive oil
- 4 eggs, beaten
- Salt and pepper to taste

Directions:

1. Preheat the air fryer for 5 minutes. In a mixing bowl, combine the eggs, coconut milk, olive oil, and butter until well-combined.
2. Add the spinach and season with salt and pepper to taste. Pour all ingredients in a baking dish that will fit in the air fryer. Bake at 3500F for 15 minutes

Nutrition:
Calories 310 Carbs 3.6g
Protein 13.6g Fat 26.8g

Caesar Marinated Grilled Chicken
Basic Recipe
Preparation Time: 5 minutes
Cooking Time: 20 minutes
Serving: 3
Ingredients:

- ¼ cup crouton

- 1 teaspoon lemon zest. Form into ovals, skewer and grill.
- 1/2 cup Parmesan
- 1/4 cup breadcrumbs
- 1-pound ground chicken
- 2 tablespoons Caesar dressing and more for drizzling
- 2-4 romaine leaves

Directions:

1. In a shallow dish, mix well chicken, 2 tablespoons Caesar dressing, parmesan, and breadcrumbs. Mix well with hands. Form into 1-inch oval patties.
2. Thread chicken pieces in skewers. Place on skewer rack in air fryer.
3. For 12 minutes, cook it on 360oF. Turnover skewers halfway through cooking time. If needed, cook in batches.
4. Serve and enjoy on a bed of lettuce and sprinkle with croutons and extra dressing.

Nutrition:
Calories 339
Carbs 9.5g
Protein 32.6g
Fat 18.9g

Cheese Stuffed Chicken
Basic Recipe
Preparation Time: 5 minutes
Cooking Time: 25 minutes
Serving: 4
Ingredients:

- 1 tablespoon creole seasoning
- 1 tablespoon olive oil
- 1 teaspoon garlic powder
- 1 teaspoon onion powder

- 4 chicken breasts, butterflied and pounded
- 4 slices Colby cheese
- 4 slices pepper jack cheese

Directions:

1. Preheat the air fryer to 3900F.
2. Place the grill pan accessory in the air fryer.
3. Create the dry rub by mixing in a bowl the creole seasoning, garlic powder, and onion powder. Season it with salt and pepper if desired.
4. Rub the seasoning on to the chicken.
5. Place the chicken on a working surface and place a slice each of pepper jack and Colby cheese.
6. Fold the chicken and secure the edges with toothpicks.
7. Brush chicken with olive oil.
8. Grill for 30 minutes and make sure to flip the meat every 10 minutes

Nutrition:
Calories 727
Carbs 5.4 g
Protein 73.1g
Fat 45.9g

Cheeseburger Egg Rolls
Basic Recipe
Preparation Time: 10 minutes
Cooking Time: 7 minutes
Servings: 6
Ingredients:

- 6 egg roll wrappers
- 6 chopped dill pickle chips
- 1 tbsp. yellow mustard
- 3 tbsp. cream cheese
- 3 tbsp. shredded cheddar cheese

- ½ C. chopped onion
- ½ C. chopped bell pepper
- ¼ tsp. onion powder
- ¼ tsp. garlic powder
- 8 ounces of raw lean ground beef

Directions:

1. In a skillet, add seasonings, beef, onion, and bell pepper. Stir and crumble beef till fully cooked, and vegetables are soft.
2. Take skillet off the heat and add cream cheese, mustard, and cheddar cheese, stirring till melted.
3. Pour beef mixture into a bowl and fold in pickles.
4. Lay out egg wrappers and place 1/6th of beef mixture into each one. Moisten egg roll wrapper edges with water. Fold sides to the middle and seal with water.
5. Repeat with all other egg rolls.
6. Place rolls into air fryer, one batch at a time.
7. Pour into the Oven rack/basket. Place the Rack on the middle-shelf of the Air Fryer Oven. Set temperature to 392°F, and set time to 7 minutes

Nutrition:
Calories 153 Cal Fat 4 g
Carbs 0 g Protein 12 g

Air Fried Grilled Steak

Basic Recipe
Preparation Time: 5 minutes
Cooking Time: 45 minutes
Servings: 2
Ingredients:

- 2 top sirloin steaks
- 3 tablespoons butter, melted

- 3 tablespoons olive oil
- Salt and pepper to taste

Directions:

1. Preheat the Air Fryer Oven for 5 minutes. Season the sirloin steaks with olive oil, salt and pepper.
2. Place the beef in the air fryer basket.
3. Cook for 45 minutes at 350°F.
4. Once cooked, serve with butter.

Nutrition:
Calories 1536
Fat 123.7 g
Carbs 0 g
Protein 103.4 g

Meat

Pork Satay
Preparation Time: 15 minutes
Cooking Time: 9-14 minutes
Servings: 4
Ingredients:

- 1 (1-pound) pork tenderloin, cut into 1½-inch cubes
- ¼ cup minced onion
- 2 garlic cloves, minced
- 1 jalapeño pepper, minced
- 2 tablespoons freshly squeezed lime juice
- 2 tablespoons coconut milk
- 2 tablespoons unsalted peanut butter
- 2 teaspoons curry powder

Directions:

1. In a medium bowl, mix the pork, onion, garlic, jalapeño, lime juice, coconut milk, peanut butter, and curry powder until well combined. Let stand for 10 minutes at room temperature.

2. With a slotted spoon, remove the pork from the marinade. Reserve the marinade.

3. Thread the pork onto about 8 bamboo (see Tip, here) or metal skewers. Grill for 9 to 14 minutes, brushing once with the reserved marinade, until the pork reaches at least 145°F on a meat thermometer. Discard any remaining marinade. Serve immediately.

Nutrition:
Calories: 194
Fat: 7g
Saturated Fat: 3g
Protein: 25g
Carbohydrates: 7g
Sodium: 65mg
Fiber: 1g
Sugar: 3g

Pork Burgers With Red Cabbage Salad

Preparation Time: 20 minutes
Cooking Time: 7-9 minutes
Servings: 4
Ingredients:

- ½ cup Greek yogurt
- 2 tablespoons low-sodium mustard, divided
- 1 tablespoon lemon juice
- ¼ cup sliced red cabbage
- ¼ cup grated carrots
- 1-pound lean ground pork
- ½ teaspoon paprika
- 1 cup mixed baby lettuce greens
- 8 small low-sodium whole-wheat sandwich buns, cut in half

Directions:

1. In a small bowl, combine the yogurt, 1 tablespoon mustard, lemon juice, cabbage, and carrots; mix and refrigerate.

2. In a medium bowl, combine the pork, remaining 1 tablespoon mustard, and paprika. Form into 8 small patties.

3. Put the sliders into the air fryer basket. Grill for 7 to 9 minutes, or until the sliders register 165°F as tested with a meat thermometer.

4. Assemble the burgers by placing some of the lettuce greens on a bun bottom. Top with cabbage mixture. Add the bun top and serve immediately.

Nutrition:
Calories: 472
Fat 15g
 Saturated Fat: 0g
Protein: 35g
Carbohydrates: 51g
Sodium 138mg
Sugar 8g
Fiber 8g

Crispy Mustard Pork Tenderloin

Preparation Time: 10 minutes
Cooking Time: 12-16 minutes
Servings: 4
Ingredients:

- 3 tablespoons low-sodium grainy mustard
- 2 teaspoons olive oil
- ¼ teaspoon dry mustard powder
- 1 (1-pound) pork tenderloin, silverskin and excess fat trimmed and discarded (see Tip, here)
- 2 slices low-sodium whole-wheat bread, crumbled
- ¼ cup ground walnuts (see Tip)
- 2 tablespoons glucomannan

Directions:
1. In a small bowl, stir together the mustard, olive oil, and mustard powder. Spread this mixture over the pork.
2. On a plate, mix the bread crumbs, walnuts, and glucomannan. Dip the mustard-coated pork into the crumb-mixture to coat.
3. Air-fry the pork for 12 to 16 minutes, or until it registers at least 145°F on a meat thermometer. Slice to serve.

Nutrition:
Calories: 239
 Fat: 9g
Saturated Fat: 2g
Protein: 26g
Carbohydrates: 15g
Sodium: 118m
Fiber: 2g
Sugar: 3g

<u>Fish</u>

Mayo Cheese Crust Salmon
Preparation Time: 10 minutes
Cooking Time: 14 minutes
Servings: 4
Ingredients:

- 4 salmon fillets
- 2 teaspoon Italian seasoning
- 2 tablespoon parmesan cheese, grated
- 2 tablespoon crushed pork rind
- 4 tablespoon mayonnaise

Directions:

1. Spread mayonnaise on top of fish fillets. Sprinkle with cheese, Italian seasoning, and crushed pork rind.
2. Place the cooking tray in the air fryer basket. Line air fryer basket with parchment paper.
3. Select Bake mode.
4. Set time to 14 minutes and temperature 375 F then press START.
5. The air fryer display will prompt you to ADD FOOD once the temperature is reached then place fish fillets in the air fryer basket.
6. Serve and enjoy.

Nutrition:
Calories 349
Fat 19.7 g
Carbohydrates 3.9 g
Sugar 1.1 g
Protein 40.1 g
Cholesterol 96 mg

Cod with Vegetables
Preparation Time: 10 minutes
Cooking Time: 15 minutes
Servings: 4
Ingredients:

- 1 lb cod fillets
- 1/2 teaspoon paprika
- 1/4 cup olive oil
- 1/4 cup lemon juice
- 8 oz asparagus, chopped
- 3 cups broccoli, chopped
- 1/2 teaspoon lemon pepper seasoning
- 1 teaspoon salt

Directions:

1. In a small bowl, mix together lemon juice, paprika, olive oil, lemon pepper seasoning, and salt.
2. Place the cooking tray in the air fryer basket. Line air fryer basket with parchment paper.
3. Select Bake mode.
4. Set time to 15 minutes and temperature 400 F then press START.
5. The air fryer display will prompt you to ADD FOOD once the temperature is reached.
6. Then place fish fillets in the middle of the parchment paper in the air fryer basket. Place broccoli and asparagus around the fish fillets.
7. Pour lemon juice mixture over the fish fillets.
8. Serve and enjoy.

Nutrition:
Calories 239 Fat 14.1 g
Carbohydrates 7.4 g Sugar 2.6 g
Protein 23.6 g Cholesterol 56 mg

Juicy Baked Halibut

Preparation Time: 10 minutes
Cooking Time: 12 minutes
Servings: 4
Ingredients:

- 1 lb halibut fillets
- 1/4 teaspoon garlic powder
- 1/4 teaspoon paprika
- 1/4 teaspoon pepper
- 1/4 cup olive oil
- 1 lemon juice
- 1/2 teaspoon salt

Directions:

1. In a small bowl, mix together olive oil, lemon juice, pepper, paprika, garlic powder, and salt.
2. Brush olive oil mixture over fish fillets.
3. Place the cooking tray in the air fryer basket. Line air fryer basket with parchment paper.
4. Select Bake mode.
5. Set time to 12 minutes and temperature 400 F then press START.
6. The air fryer display will prompt you to ADD FOOD once the temperature is reached then place fish fillets in the air fryer basket.
7. Serve and enjoy.

Nutrition:
Calories 272 Fat 15.4 g
Carbohydrates 0.5 g Sugar 0.3 g
Protein 30.8 g Cholesterol 53 mg

<u>Vegetable</u>

Healthy Eggplant Salad

Preparation Time: 10 minutes

Cooking Time: 25 minutes

Serve: 6

Ingredients:

- 1 lb eggplant, cut into slices
- 1/4 cup olive oil

- 1 tbsp fresh lemon juice
- 1 tbsp parsley, chopped
- 1 tbsp cilantro, chopped
- 1/2 tsp paprika
- 1 tsp ground cumin
- 1 garlic clove, grated
- 1/2 tsp salt

Directions:

1. Brush eggplant slices with 2 tbsp oil.
2. Place eggplant slices onto a cooking tray.
3. Select BAKE mode, then set the temperature to 400 F and the time to 25 minutes, then press start.
4. When the display shows Add Food then place the cooking tray in the vortex plus air fryer oven.
5. In a bowl, mix together the remaining ingredients and pour over eggplant slices.
6. Mix well and serve.

Nutrition:

Calories 94

Fat 8.7 g

Carbohydrates 5 g

Sugar 2.4 g

Protein 0.9 g

Cholesterol 0 mg

Spiced Green Beans

Preparation Time: 10 minutes
Cooking Time: 10 minutes
Servings: 2
Ingredients:

- 2 cups green beans
- 1/8 teaspoon cayenne pepper
- 1/8 teaspoon ground allspice
- 1/4 teaspoon ground cinnamon
- 1/2 teaspoon dried oregano
- 2 tablespoon olive oil
- 1/4 teaspoon ground coriander
- 1/4 teaspoon ground cumin
- 1/2 teaspoon salt

Directions:

1. Add all ingredients into the mixing bowl and toss well.
2. Select Air Fry mode.
3. Set time to 10 minutes and temperature 370 F then press START.
4. The air fryer display will prompt you to ADD FOOD once the temperature is reached then add green beans in the air fryer basket. Stir Halfway through.
5. Serve and enjoy.

Nutrition:
Calories 158 Fat 14.3 g
Carbohydrates 8.6 g Sugar 1.6 g
Protein 2.1 g Cholesterol 0 mg

Roasted Squash

Preparation Time: 10 minutes
Cooking Time: 60 minutes
Servings: 4

Ingredients:

- 2 lbs summer squash, cut into 1-inch pieces
- 1/8 teaspoon garlic powder
- 3 tablespoon olive oil
- 1 large lemon
- 1/8 teaspoon paprika
- 1/8 teaspoon pepper
- Pepper
- Salt

Directions:

1. Place squash pieces into the baking dish and drizzle with olive oil.
2. Season with paprika, pepper, and garlic powder.
3. Squeeze lemon juice over the squash.
4. Select Bake mode.
5. Set time to 60 minutes and temperature 400 F then press START.
6. The air fryer display will prompt you to ADD FOOD once the temperature is reached then place the baking dish in the air fryer basket.
7. Serve and enjoy.

Nutrition:
Calories 138 Fat 11.2 g
Carbohydrates 10.3 g Sugar 8.4 g
Protein 2.5 g Cholesterol 0 mg

Snacks

Oregano Chicken Wings
Preparation time: 15 minutes
Cooking time: 12 minutes
Servings: 5
Ingredients:

- 1 teaspoon stevia extract
- 1 teaspoon salt
- 1-pound chicken wings
- 1 teaspoon paprika
- 1 teaspoon dried oregano
- 1 tablespoon olive oil

Directions:

1. Combine the salt, paprika, and dried oregano in a bowl and stir.
2. Coat the chicken wings with the spices.
3. Sprinkle the chicken wings with the stevia extract.
4. Preheat the air fryer to 400 F.
5. Place the Prepared chicken wings in the air fryer rack and drizzle them with olive oil.
6. Cook for 12 minutes.
7. Remove and place them on a paper towel to drain any excess grease.

Nutrition:
calories 199,
fat 9.6,
fiber 0.3,
carbs 0.4,
protein 26.3

Keto French Fries
Preparation time: 10 minutes
Cooking time: 15 minutes
Servings: 6
Ingredients:

- 2 sweet dumpling squashes
- 1 teaspoon paprika
- ¼ teaspoon ground white pepper
- ¼ teaspoon salt

- 1 tablespoon olive oil

Directions:

1. Peel the sweet dumpling squash and cut it into the strips.

2. Cover the air fryer basket tray with the parchment and place the sweet dumpling squash strips there.

3. Then sprinkle the sweet dumpling squash strips with the ground white pepper, paprika, and salt.

4. Spray the sweet dumpling squash strips with the olive oil.

5. Preheat the air fryer to 365 F.

6. Cook the sweet dumpling squash fries for 15 minutes. The time can be less or more — depends on the size of the sweet dumpling squash strips.

7. Then transfer the fries to the serving plate and chill them.

8. Enjoy!

Nutrition:
calories 30,
fat 2.4,
fiber 0.7,
carbs 2.3,
protein 0.2

Paprika Zucchini Chips

Preparation time: 8 minutes
Cooking time: 13 minutes
Servings: 5
Ingredients:

- 2 zucchinis
- 1 teaspoon olive oil
- ½ teaspoon salt
- 1 teaspoon paprika

Directions:

1. Wash the zucchini carefully and slice into chips pieces.

2. Preheat the air fryer to 370 F.

3. Sprinkle the zucchini slices with salt and paprika.

4. Place the zucchini slices in the air fryer rack.

5. Drizzle the zucchini slices with olive oil.

6. Cook for 13 minutes.

7. Turn the zucchini over if required.

8. When the zucchini chips are cooked let them cool.

9. Serve or keep them in a paper bag.

Nutrition:
calories 22,
fat 1.1,
fiber 1,
carbs 2.9,
protein 1

Paprika Avocado Fries

Preparation time: 10 minutes
Cooking time: 10 minutes
Servings: 4
Ingredients:

- 1 avocado, pitted
- ½ teaspoon salt
- 1 teaspoon ground black pepper
- ½ teaspoon paprika
- 1 egg
- 1 tablespoon coconut flour
- 1 teaspoon olive oil

Directions:

1. Peel the avocado and cut it into thick strips.

2. Crack the egg in a bowl and whisk.

3. Combine the salt, ground black pepper, paprika, and coconut flour.

4. Coat the avocado strips with the whisked egg.

5. Coat each avocado strip in the spice mixture.

6. Place the avocado strips in the air fryer rack and drizzle them with olive oil.

7. Set the air fryer to 390 F and cook the avocado fries for 10 minutes.

8. Shake the avocado fries gently and cook them for 5 minutes more.

Nutrition:
calories 164,
fat 14.4,
fiber 4.3,
carbs 6.5,
protein 2.4

Dessert

Vanilla Shortcake
Preparation time: 15 minutes
Cooking time: 30 minutes
Servings: 4
Ingredients:
- 3 eggs, beaten
- ½ cup almond flour
- ½ teaspoon baking powder
- 2 teaspoons swerve
- 1 teaspoon vanilla extract
- ½ cup coconut cream
- Cooking spray

Directions:

1. Spray the air fryer basket with cooking spray.

2. Then mix eggs with almond flour, baking powder, swerve, vanilla extract, and coconut cream.

3. When the mixture is smooth, pour it in the air fryer basket and flatten gently with the help of the spatula.

4. Cook the shortcake at 355F for 30 minutes.

Nutrition:
calories 140,
fat 12.2,
fiber 1.1,
carbs 3.1,
protein 5.6

Raspberry Cream
Preparation Time: 10 minutes
Cooking time: 20 minutes
Servings: 6
Ingredients:
- ½ cup raspberries
- 1 tablespoon lime juice
- 2 tablespoons water
- 3 tablespoons Erythritol
- ¼ teaspoon ground cinnamon

Directions:

1. Blend the raspberries and mix with lime juice, water, Erythritol, and ground cinnamon.

2. Pour the mixture in the air fryer and cook at 345F for 20 minutes.

Nutrition:
calories 6, fat 0.1,
fiber 0.7, carbs 1.5, protein 0.1

Coconut Hand Pies
Preparation time: 20 minutes
Cooking time: 26 minutes
Servings: 6

Ingredients:

- 8 oz coconut flour
- 1 teaspoon vanilla extract
- 2 tablespoons Swerve
- 2 eggs, beaten
- 1 tablespoon almond butter, melted
- 1 tablespoon almond meal
- 2 tablespoons coconut shred
- Cooking spray

Directions:

1. Mix coconut flour with vanilla extract, Swerve, eggs, almond butter, and almond meal.
2. Knead the dough and roll it up.
3. Cut the dough into squares and sprinkle with coconut shred.
4. Fold the squares into the shape of pies and put in the air fryer basket.
5. Sprinkle the pies with cooking spray and cook at 345F for 13 minutes per side.

Nutrition:
calories 128,
fat 6.5,
fiber 7.1,
carbs 11.7,
protein 5.1

Milk Pie

Preparation Time: 10 minutes
Cooking time: 20 minutes
Servings: 8
Ingredients:

- 2 egg, beaten
- 3 tablespoons Erythritol
- 3 tablespoons butter, melted
- ¼ cup organic almond milk
- 4 tablespoons coconut flour
- ½ teaspoon baking powder

Directions:

1. Put all ingredients in the mixer bowl and blend until smooth.
2. Pour the mixture in the air fryer basket and cook at 365F for 20 minutes.

Nutrition:
calories 73,
fat 6.1,
fiber 1.3,
carbs 2.6,
protein 2.2

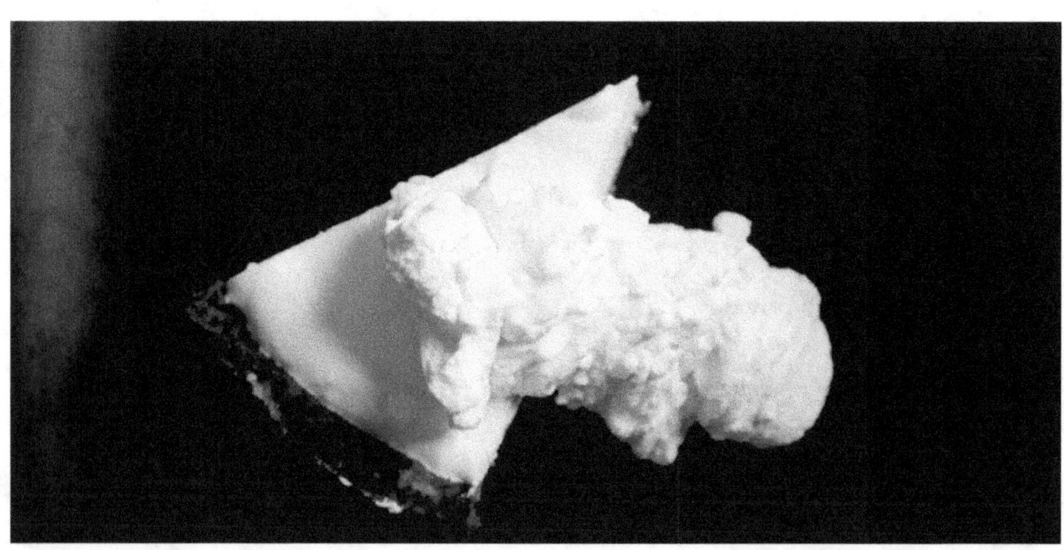

CHAPTER 10:

August

Lunch

Chicken Coconut Poppers
Preparation time: 10 minutes
Cooking time: 10 minutes
Servings: 6
Ingredients:

- ½ cup coconut flour
- 1 teaspoon chili flakes
- 1 teaspoon ground black pepper
- 1 teaspoon garlic powder
- 11 oz. chicken breast, boneless, skinless
- 1 tablespoon olive oil

Directions:

1. Cut the chicken breast into medium cubes and put them in a large bowl.
2. Sprinkle the chicken cubes with the chili flakes, ground black pepper, garlic powder, and stir them well using your hands.
3. After this, sprinkle the chicken cubes with the almond flour.
4. Shake the bowl with the chicken cubes gently to coat the meat.
5. Preheat the air fryer to 365 F.
6. Grease the air fryer basket tray with the olive oil.
7. Place the chicken cubes inside.
8. Cook the chicken poppers for 10 minutes.
9. Turn the chicken poppers over after 5 minutes of cooking.
10. Allow the cooked chicken poppers to cool before serving.

Nutrition:
calories 123,
fat 4.6,
fiber 3.9,
carbs 6.9,
protein 13.2

Paprika Pulled Pork
Preparation time: 15 minutes
Cooking time: 20 minutes
Servings: 4
Ingredients:

- 1 tablespoon chili flakes
- 1 teaspoon ground black pepper
- ½ teaspoon paprika
- 1 teaspoon cayenne pepper
- 1/3 cup cream
- 1 teaspoon kosher salt
- 1-pound pork tenderloin

- 1 teaspoon ground thyme
- 4 cup chicken stock
- 1 teaspoon butter

Directions:

1. Pour the chicken stock into the air fryer basket tray.
2. Add the pork steak and sprinkle the mixture with the chili flakes, ground black pepper, paprika, cayenne pepper, and kosher salt.
3. Preheat the air fryer to 370 F and cook the meat for 20 minutes.
4. Strain the liquid and shred the meat with 2 forks.
5. Then add the butter and cream and mix it.
6. Cook the pulled pork for 4 minutes more at 360 F.
7. When the pulled pork is cooked allow to rest briefly.

Nutrition:
calories 198,
fat 6.8,
fiber 0.5,
carbs 2.3,
protein 30.7

Paprika Whole Chicken

Preparation time: 15 minutes
Cooking time: 75 minutes
Servings: 12
Ingredients:

- 6-pound whole chicken
- 1 teaspoon kosher salt
- 1 teaspoon ground black pepper
- 1 teaspoon ground paprika
- 1 tablespoon minced garlic
- 3 tablespoon butter

- 1 teaspoon olive oil
- ¼ cup water
- 3 oz chive stems

Directions:

1. Rub the whole chicken with the kosher salt and ground black pepper inside and outside.
2. Sprinkle it with the ground paprika and minced garlic.
3. Dice the chives.
4. Put the diced chives inside the whole chicken.
5. Then add the butter.
6. Rub the chicken with olive oil.
7. Preheat the air fryer to 360 F and pour water in the air fryer basket.
8. Place the chicken on the rack inside the air fryer.
9. Cook the chicken for 75 minutes.
10. When the chicken is cooked it should have slightly crunchy skin.
11. Cut the cooked chicken into the servings.

Nutrition:
calories 464, fat 20.1,
fiber 0.2, carbs 0.9, protein 65.8

Pork Almond Bites

Preparation time: 10 minutes
Cooking time: 14 minutes
Servings: 6
Ingredients:

- 1-pound pork tenderloin
- 2 eggs
- 1 teaspoon butter
- ¼ cup almond flour

- 1 teaspoon kosher salt
- 1 teaspoon paprika
- 1 teaspoon ground coriander
- ½ teaspoon lemon zest

Directions:
1. Chop the pork tenderloin into the large cubes.
2. Sprinkle the pork cubes with the kosher salt, paprika, ground coriander, and lemon zest.
3. Mix the meat gently.
4. Crack the egg into a bowl and whisk it.
5. Coat the meat cubes with the egg mixture and then the almond flour.
6. Preheat the air fryer to 365 F.
7. Put the butter in the air fryer basket tray and then place the pork bites inside.
8. Cook the pork bites for 14 minutes.
9. Turn the pork bites over after 7 minutes of cooking.
10. When the pork bites are cooked – serve them hot.

Nutrition:
calories 142, fat 5.4,
fiber 0.3, carbs 0.6, protein 21.9

Pandan Coconut Chicken

Preparation time: 20 minutes
Cooking time: 10 minutes
Servings: 4
Ingredients:

- 15oz. chicken
- 1 pandan leaf
- 3 oz chive stems, diced
- 1 teaspoon minced garlic
- 1 teaspoon chili flakes
- 1 teaspoon stevia
- 1 teaspoon ground black pepper
- 1 teaspoon turmeric
- 1 tablespoon butter
- ¼ cup coconut milk
- 1 tablespoon chives powder

Directions:
1. Cut the chicken into 4 big cubes.
2. Put the chicken cubes in a large bowl.
3. Sprinkle the chicken with the minced garlic, diced chives, chili flakes, stevia, ground black pepper, chives powder, and turmeric.
4. Mix the meat up using your hands.
5. Cut the pandan leaf into 4 parts.
6. Wrap the chicken cubes into the pandan leaf.
7. Pour the coconut milk into a bowl with the wrapped chicken and leave it for 10 minutes.
8. Preheat the air fryer to 380 F.
9. Put the pandan chicken in the air fryer basket and cook for 10 minutes.
10. When the chicken is cooked – transfer to serving plates and let it chill for at least 2-3 minutes.

Nutrition:
calories 250, fat 12.6,
fiber 0.9, carbs 3.1, protein 29.9

Dinner

Juicy Cheeseburgers

Basic Recipe
Preparation Time: 5 minutes
Cooking Time: 15 minutes
Servings: 4
Ingredients:

- 1 pound 93% lean ground beef
- 1 teaspoon Worcestershire sauce
- 1 tablespoon burger seasoning
- Salt
- Pepper
- Cooking oil
- 4 slices cheese
- Buns

Directions:

1. In a large bowl, mix the ground beef, Worcestershire, burger seasoning, and salt and pepper to taste until well blended. Spray the air fryer basket with cooking oil. You will need only a quick sprits. The burgers will produce oil as they cook. Shape the mixture into 4 patties. Place the burgers in the air fryer. The burgers should fit without the need to stack, but stacking is okay if necessary.
2. Pour into the Oven rack/basket. Place the Rack on the middle-shelf of the Air Fryer Oven. Set temperature to 375°F, and set time to 8 minutes Cook for 8 minutes Open the air fryer and flip the burgers. Cook for an additional 3 to 4 minutes Check the inside of the burgers to determine if they have finished cooking. You can stick a knife or fork in the center to examine the color.
3. Top each burger with a slice of cheese. Cook for an additional minute, or until the cheese has melted
4. Serve on buns with any additional toppings of your choice.

Nutrition:
Calories 566 Cal
Fat 39 g
Carbs 0 g
Protein 29 g

Spicy Thai Beef Stir-Fry

Basic Recipe
Preparation Time: 15 minutes
Cooking Time: 9 minutes
Servings: 4
Ingredients:

- 1-pound sirloin steaks, thinly sliced
- 2 tablespoons lime juice, divided
- ⅓Cup crunchy peanut butter
- ½ cup beef broth
- 1 tablespoon olive oil
- 1½ cups broccoli florets
- 2 cloves garlic, sliced
- 1 to 2 red chili peppers, sliced

Directions:

1. In a medium bowl, combine the steak with 1 tablespoon of the lime juice. Set aside.
2. Combine the peanut butter and beef broth in a small bowl and mix well. Dry out the beef and add the juice from the bowl into the peanut butter mixture.
3. In a 6-inch metal bowl, combine the olive oil, steak, and broccoli.

4. Pour into the Oven rack/basket. Place the Rack on the middle-shelf of the Air Fryer Oven. Set temperature to 375°F, and set time to 4 minutes Cook for 3 to 4 minutes or until the steak is almost cooked and the broccoli is crisp and tender, shaking the basket once during cooking time.

5. Add the garlic, chili peppers, and the peanut butter mixture and stir.

6. Cook for 3 to 5 minutes or until the sauce is bubbling and the broccoli is tender.

7. Serve over hot cauliflower rice.

Nutrition:
Calories 387 Cal
Fat 22 g
Carbs 0 g
Protein 42 g

Beef Brisket Recipe from Texas

Basic Recipe
Preparation Time: 15 minutes
Cooking Time: 1 hour and 30 minutes
Servings: 8
Ingredients:

- 1 ½ cup beef stock
- 1 bay leaf
- 1 tablespoon garlic powder
- 1 tablespoon onion powder
- 2 pounds beef brisket, trimmed
- 2 tablespoons chili powder
- 2 teaspoons dry mustard
- 4 tablespoons olive oil
- Salt and pepper to taste

Directions:

1. Preheat the Air Fryer Oven for 5 minutes Place all ingredients in a deep baking dish that will fit in the air fryer.

2. Bake it for 1 hour and 30 minutes at 400°F.

3. Stir the beef every after 30 minutes to soak in the sauce.

Nutrition:
Calories 306 Cal
Fat 24.1 g
Carbs 0 g
Protein 18.3 g

Copycat Taco Bell Crunch Wraps

Basic Recipe
Preparation Time: 10 minutes
Cooking Time: 2 minutes
Servings: 6
Ingredients:

- 6 wheat tostadas
- 2 C. sour cream
- 2 C. Mexican blend cheese
- 2 C. shredded lettuce
- 12 ounces low-sodium nacho cheese
- 6 12-inch wheat tortillas
- 1 1/3 C. water
- 2 packets low-sodium taco seasoning
- 2 pounds of lean ground beef

Directions:

1. Ensure your air fryer is preheated to 400 degrees.

2. Make beef according to taco seasoning packets.

3. Place 2/3 C. prepared beef, 4 tbsp. cheese, 1 tostada, 1/3 C. sour cream, 1/3 C. lettuce, and 1/3 C. cheese on each tortilla.

4. Fold up tortillas edges and repeat with remaining ingredients.

5. Lay the folded sides of tortillas down into the air fryer and spray with olive oil.
6. Set temperature to 400°F, and set time to 2 minutes Cook 2 minutes till browned.

Nutrition:
Calories 311 Cal
Fat 9 g
Carbs 0 g
Protein 22 g

Air Fryer Beef Casserole

Basic Recipe
Preparation Time: 5 minutes
Cooking Time: 30 minutes
Servings: 4
Ingredients:

- 1 green bell pepper, seeded and chopped
- 1 onion, chopped
- 1-pound ground beef
- 3 cloves of garlic, minced
- 3 tablespoons olive oil
- 6 cups eggs, beaten
- Salt and pepper to taste

Directions:
1. Preheat the Air Fryer Oven for 5 minutes
2. In a baking dish that will fit in the air fryer, mix the ground beef, onion, garlic, olive oil, and bell pepper. Season it with salt and pepper to taste.
3. Pour in the beaten eggs and give a good stir.
4. Place the dish with the beef and egg mixture in the air fryer.
5. Pour into the Oven rack/basket. Place the Rack on the middle-shelf of the Air Fryer Oven. Set

temperature to 325°F, and set time to 30 minutes. Bake it for 30 minutes

Nutrition:
Calories 1520 Cal
Fat 125.11 g
Carbs 0 g
Protein 87.9 g

Meat Lovers' Pizza

Intermediate Recipe
Preparation Time: 10 minutes
Cooking Time: 12 minutes
Servings: 2
Ingredients:

- 1 pre-prepared 7-inch pizza pie crust, defrosted if necessary
- 1/3 cup of marinara sauce
- 2 ounces of grilled steak, sliced into bite-sized pieces
- 2 ounces of salami, sliced fine
- 2 ounces of pepperoni, sliced fine
- ¼ cup of American cheese
- ¼ cup of shredded mozzarella cheese

Directions:
1. Preheat the Air Fryer Oven to 350 degrees. Lay the pizza dough flat on a sheet of parchment paper or tin foil, cut large enough to hold the entire pie crust, but small enough that it will leave the edges of the air frying basket uncovered to allow for air circulation. Using a fork, stab the pizza dough several times across the surface – piercing the pie crust will allow air to circulate throughout the crust and ensure even cooking. With a deep soup spoon, ladle the marinara sauce onto the pizza

dough, and spread evenly in expanding circles over the surface of the pie-crust. Be sure to leave at least ½ inch of bare dough around the edges, to ensure that extra-crispy crunchy first bite of the crust! Distribute the pieces of steak and the slices of salami and pepperoni evenly over the sauce-covered dough, then sprinkle the cheese in an even layer on top.

2. Set the air fryer timer to 12 minutes, and place the pizza with foil or paper on the fryer's basket surface. Again, be sure to leave the edges of the basket uncovered to allow for proper air circulation, and don't let your bare fingers touch the hot surface. After 12 minutes, when the Air Fryer Oven shuts off, the cheese should be perfectly melted and lightly crisped, and the pie crust should be golden brown. Using a spatula – or two, if necessary, remove the pizza from the air fryer basket and set on a serving plate. Wait a few minutes until the pie is cool enough to handle, then cut into slices and serve.

Nutrition:
Calories 390 Cal
Fat 21 g
Carbs 34 g
Fiber 3 g

<u>Meat</u>

Pork Tenderloin
Preparation Time: 10 minutes
Cooking Time: 14-19 minutes

Servings: 4
Ingredients:
- 1 (1-pound) pork tenderloin, cut into 4 pieces
- 3 celery stalks, sliced
- 1 onion, sliced
- ½ teaspoon dried marjoram

Directions:
1. Rub each piece of pork with the olive oil.
2. In a medium metal bowl, mix the pork, celery, onion, marjoram, and apple juice.
3. Place the bowl into the air fryer and roast for 14 to 19 minutes, or until the pork reaches at least 145°F on a meat thermometer and the vegetables are tender. Stir once during cooking. Serve immediately.

Nutrition:
Calories: 213
Fat: 5g
Saturated Fat: 1g
Protein: 24g
Carbohydrates: 20g
Sodium: 88mg
Fiber: 3g
Sugar: 15g

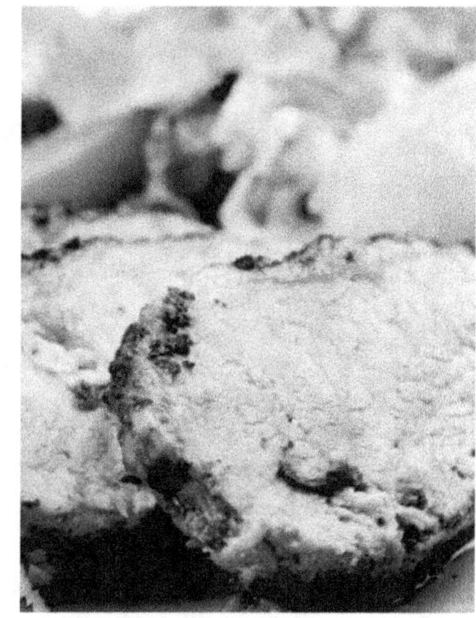

Espresso-Grilled Pork Tenderloin

Preparation Time: 15 minutes
Cooking Time: 9-11 minutes
Servings: 4
Ingredients:

- 1 tablespoon packed brown sugar
- 2 teaspoons espresso powder
- 1 teaspoon ground paprika
- ½ teaspoon dried marjoram
- 1 tablespoon honey
- 1 tablespoon freshly squeezed lemon juice
- 2 teaspoons olive oil
- 1 (1-pound) pork tenderloin

Directions:

1. In a small bowl, mix the brown sugar, espresso powder, paprika, and marjoram.
2. Stir in the honey, lemon juice, and olive oil until well mixed.
3. Spread the honey mixture over the pork and let stand for 10 minutes at room temperature.
4. Roast the tenderloin in the air fryer basket for 9 to 11 minutes, or until the pork registers at least 145°F on a meat thermometer. Slice the meat to serve.

Nutrition:
Calories: 177
Fat: 5g
Saturated Fat: 1g
Protein: 23g
Carbohydrates: 10g
Sodium: 61mg
Fiber: 1g
 Sugar: 8g

Pork And Carrots

Preparation Time: 5 minutes
Cooking Time: 25 minutes
Servings: 4
Ingredients:

- 2 cups creamer carrots, rinsed and dried
- 2 teaspoons olive oil (see Tip)
- 1 (1-pound) pork tenderloin, cut into 1-inch cubes
- 1 onion, chopped
- 1 red bell pepper, chopped
- 2 garlic cloves, minced
- ½ teaspoon dried oregano
- 2 tablespoons low-sodium chicken broth

Directions:

1. In a medium bowl, toss the carrots and olive oil to coat.
2. Transfer the carrots to the air fryer basket. Roast for 15 minutes.
3. In a medium metal bowl, mix the carrots, pork, onion, red bell pepper, garlic, and oregano.
4. Drizzle with the chicken broth. Put the bowl in the air fryer basket. Roast for about 10 minutes more, shaking the basket once during cooking, until the pork reaches at least 145°F on a meat thermometer and the carrots are tender. Serve immediately.

Nutrition:
Calories: 235 Fat: 5g
Saturated Fat: 1g
Protein: 26g
Carbohydrates: 22g
Sodium: 66mg
Fiber: 3g
Sugar: 4g

<u>Fish</u>

Delicious Crab Cakes

Preparation Time: 10 minutes
Cooking Time: 20 minutes
Servings: 4
Ingredients:

- 1 lb lump crab meat
- 1 tablespoon butter, melted
- 1/2 teaspoon old bay seasoning
- 1 tablespoon parsley, chopped
- 1 teaspoon garlic powder
- 1 teaspoon onion powder
- 1/4 cup parmesan cheese
- 1 egg yolk, lightly beaten
- 1 egg, lightly beaten
- 2 teaspoon Dijon mustard
- 1/4 cup mayonnaise

Directions:

1. Add all ingredients except melted butter into the mixing bowl and mix until well combined.
2. Make 4 equal shapes of patties from the mixture.
3. Place the cooking tray in the air fryer basket. Line air fryer basket with parchment paper.
4. Select Bake mode.
5. Set time to 20 minutes and temperature 400 F then press START.
6. The air fryer display will prompt you to ADD FOOD once the temperature is reached then place patties in the air fryer basket and drizzle with melted butter.
7. Serve and enjoy.

Nutrition:
Calories 247 Fat 22.4 g Carbohydrates 7.3 g Sugar 1.5 g Protein 23.7 g Cholesterol 179 mg

Lemon Garlic Shrimp

Preparation Time: 10 minutes
Cooking Time: 14 minutes
Servings: 3
Ingredients:

- 1 lb shrimp, peeled & deveined
- 1/4 teaspoon garlic powder
- 1 tablespoon olive oil
- 1/2 lemon
- Pepper
- Salt

Directions:

1. In a mixing bowl, toss shrimp with garlic powder, olive oil, pepper, and salt.
2. Place the cooking tray in the air fryer basket.
3. Select Air Fry mode.
4. Set time to 14 minutes and temperature 400 F then press START.
5. The air fryer display will prompt you to ADD FOOD once the temperature is reached then add shrimp in the air fryer basket. Shake basket halfway through.
6. Squeeze lemon juice over shrimp and serve.

Nutrition:
Calories 223 Fat 7.3 g
Carbohydrates 3.4 g Sugar 0.3 g
Protein 34.6 g
Cholesterol 318 mg

Simple Salmon Patties

Preparation Time: 10 minutes
Cooking Time: 14 minutes
Servings: 4
Ingredients:

- 2 eggs, lightly beaten
- 2 oz salmon, cooked and flaked
- 1/4 teaspoon paprika
- 1/8 teaspoon pepper
- 1/3 cup parsley, chopped
- 2 garlic cloves, minced
- 1/4 cup onion, diced
- 2/3 cup almond flour
- Pinch of salt

Directions:

1. Add all ingredients into the mixing bowl and mix until well combined.
2. Make the equal shape of patties from the mixture.
3. Place the cooking tray in the air fryer basket. Line air fryer basket with parchment paper.
4. Select Air Fry mode.
5. Set time to 14 minutes and temperature 380 F then press START.
6. The air fryer display will prompt you to ADD FOOD once the temperature is reached then place patties in the air fryer basket.
7. Turn patties halfway through.
8. Serve and enjoy.

Nutrition:
Calories 84 Fat 5.5 g
Carbohydrates 2.8 g
Sugar 0.7 g Protein 6.9 g
Cholesterol 88 mg

Snacks

Eggplant Bites with Parmesan

Preparation time: 8 minutes
Cooking time: 14 minutes
Servings: 4
Ingredients:

- 1 eggplant
- ½ teaspoon turmeric
- ¼ teaspoon salt
- 4 oz. Parmesan, sliced
- 1 teaspoon olive oil

Directions:

1. Cut the eggplants into four pieces.
2. Coat the eggplant with turmeric, salt, and mix well.
3. Preheat the air fryer to 400 F.
4. Place the eggplant in the air fryer basket tray and drizzle them with olive oil.
5. Cook for 13 minutes.
6. Cover the eggplant with sliced Parmesan.
7. Cook for a further minute.
8. Transfer to a serving plate to cool slightly before serving.

Nutrition:
calories 131,
fat 7.5,
fiber 4.1,
carbs 7.9,
protein 10.3

Ginger Chicken Wings

Preparation time: 15 minutes
Cooking time: 14 minutes

Servings: 4
Ingredients:

- 1-pound chicken wings
- ½ teaspoon salt
- 1 teaspoon garlic powder
- ¼ teaspoon ground black pepper
- ¼ teaspoon cayenne pepper
- ½ teaspoon ground ginger
- 1 tablespoon mustard

Directions:

1. Place the chicken wings in a mixing bowl.
2. Coat the wings with salt, garlic powder, ground black pepper, cayenne pepper, ground ginger, and mustard.
3. Mix well.
4. Marinade for 10 minutes.
5. Preheat the air fryer to 370 F.
6. Place the chicken wings in the air fryer basket tray and cook for 14 minutes.

Nutrition:
calories 234, fat 9.3, fiber 0.6,
carbs 2.1,
protein 33.7

Lamb Chives Burgers

Preparation time: 15 minutes
Cooking time: 9 minutes
Servings: 6
Ingredients:

- 1-pound ground lamb
- 3 oz chive stems
- 1 teaspoon minced garlic
- 1 teaspoon salt
- ½ teaspoon chili pepper
- 1 teaspoon ground black pepper
- 1 large egg
- 2 tablespoon coconut flour
- 1 teaspoon olive oil

Directions:

1. Combine the ground lamb with the diced chives.
2. Stir carefully and sprinkle the mixture with minced garlic and salt.
3. Add chili pepper, ground black pepper, and coconut flour.
4. Crack the egg into the mixture and mix with your hands.
5. Place the mixture in the fridge for 10 minutes.
6. Meanwhile, preheat the air fryer to 400 F.
7. Make 6 large balls from the ground lamb mixture and flatten them to make the shape of a burger patty.
8. Place the burgers in the air fryer rack and drizzle them with olive oil.
9. Cook for 6 minutes.
10. Turn them using a spatula.
11. Cook the lamb burgers for 3 minutes.
12. Serve hot.

Nutrition:
calories 178, fat 7.4,
fiber 1.5,
carbs 3.9,
protein 22.9

Cheddar-stuffed Mushrooms

Preparation time: 10 minutes
Cooking time: 5 minutes
Servings: 7
Ingredients:

- 9 oz. mushroom tops
- 6 oz. Cheddar cheese, shredded
- 1 teaspoon dried dill
- 1 teaspoon dried parsley
- ½ teaspoon salt
- 1 tablespoon butter

Directions:

1. Remove the flesh from the mushroom tops and chop finely.
2. Combine the ground mushroom flesh with the dried dill and dried parsley.
3. Add salt and soft butter and mix.
4. Combine the mixture with the shredded cheese.
5. Stir.
6. Fill the mushroom tops with the cheese mixture.
7. Preheat the air fryer to 400 F.
8. Put the mushrooms in the air fryer rack and cook them for 5 minutes.
9. Transfer to a serving plate.

Nutrition:
calories 121,
fat 9.8,
fiber 0.4,
carbs 1.6,
protein 7.3

Vegetable

Tasty Baked Cauliflower

Preparation Time: 10 minutes
Cooking Time: 45 minutes
Servings: 2
Ingredients:

- 1/2 cauliflower head, cut into florets
- 2 tablespoon olive oil

For seasoning:

- 1/2 teaspoon garlic powder
- 1 teaspoon onion powder
- 1 tablespoon ground cayenne pepper
- 2 tablespoon ground paprika
- 1/2 teaspoon ground cumin
- 1/2 teaspoon black pepper
- 1/2 teaspoon white pepper
- 2 teaspoon salt

Directions:

1. In a large bowl, mix together all seasoning ingredients.
2. Add oil and stir well. Add cauliflower to the bowl seasoning mixture and stir well to coat.
3. Transfer the cauliflower florets into the baking dish.
4. Select Bake mode.
5. Set time to 45 minutes and temperature 400 F then press START.
6. The air fryer display will prompt you to ADD FOOD once the temperature is reached then place the baking dish in the air fryer basket.

7. Serve and enjoy.

Nutrition:
Calories 176
Fat 15.6 g
Carbohydrates 11.3 g
Sugar 3.2 g
Protein 3.1 g
Cholesterol 0 mg

Parmesan Baked Zucchini

Preparation Time: 10 minutes
Cooking Time: 35 minutes
Servings: 6
Ingredients:

- 2 1/2 lbs zucchini, cut into quarters
- 1/2 cup parmesan cheese, shredded
- 6 garlic cloves, crushed
- 1/2 teaspoon black pepper
- 1/3 cup parsley, chopped
- 1 teaspoon dried basil
- 3/4 teaspoon salt

Directions:

1. Add all ingredients except parsley into the large mixing bowl and stir well to combine.
2. Pour egg mixture into the greased baking dish.
3. Select Bake mode.
4. Set time to 35 minutes and temperature 350 F then press START.
5. The air fryer display will prompt you to ADD FOOD once the temperature is reached then place the baking dish in the air fryer basket.
6. Serve and enjoy.

Nutrition:

Calories 108
Fat 4.7 g
Carbohydrates 10.2 g
Sugar 4.6 g
Protein 9.3 g
Cholesterol 14 mg

Broccoli Nuggets

Preparation Time: 10 minutes
Cooking Time: 20 minutes
Servings: 4
Ingredients:

- 2 cups broccoli florets, cooked until soften
- 1/4 cup almond flour
- 2 egg whites
- 1 cup cheddar cheese, shredded
- 1/8 teaspoon salt

Directions:

1. Add cooked broccoli florets into the large bowl and using potato masher mash into small pieces.
2. Add remaining ingredients into the bowl and mix until well combined.
3. Make small nuggets from the broccoli mixture.
4. Select Bake mode.
5. Set time to 20 minutes and temperature 350 F then press START.
6. The air fryer display will prompt you to ADD FOOD once the temperature is reached then place broccoli nuggets in the air fryer basket.
7. Serve and enjoy.

Nutrition:

Calories 148
Fat 10.4 g
Carbohydrates 3.9 g
Sugar 1.1 g
Protein 10.5 g
Cholesterol 30 mg

Cheese Baked Broccoli
Preparation Time: 10 minutes
Cooking Time: 10 minutes
Servings: 4
Ingredients:

- 1 lb broccoli, cut into florets
- 1/2 cup mozzarella cheese, shredded
- 1/2 cup heavy cream
- 2 garlic cloves, minced
- 1/4 cup parmesan cheese, grated
- 1/2 cup gruyere cheese, shredded
- 1 tablespoon butter

Directions:
1. Melt butter in a pan over medium heat.
2. Add broccoli and season with pepper and salt.
3. Cook broccoli over medium heat for 5 minutes or until tender. Add garlic and stir for a minute.
4. Transfer broccoli into the baking dish.
5. Pour heavy cream over broccoli then top with parmesan cheese, gruyere cheese, and mozzarella cheese.
6. Select Bake mode.
7. Set time to 10 minutes and temperature 375 F then press START.
8. The air fryer display will prompt you to ADD FOOD once the temperature is reached then place the baking dish in the air fryer basket.
9. Serve and enjoy.

Nutrition:
Calories 230
Fat 16.9 g
Carbohydrates 9.2 g
Sugar 2 g
Protein 13.3 g
Cholesterol 55 mg

Dessert

Keto Hot Chocolate
Preparation time: 10 minutes
Cooking time: 7 minutes
Servings: 3
Ingredients:

- 1/4 teaspoon vanilla extract
- 2 cups organic almond milk
- 1 teaspoon coconut oil
- 1 tablespoon cocoa powder
- 2 tablespoons Erythritol

Directions:
1. Mix all ingredients in the air fryer basket.
2. Stir the mixture until smooth.
3. Cook the dessert at 375F for 7 minutes.

Nutrition:
calories 386, fat 39.9, fiber 4.1,
carbs 9.9,
protein 4

Cocoa Chia Pudding

Preparation Time: 40 minutes
Cooking time: 10 minutes
Servings: 3
Ingredients:

- 3 tablespoons chia seeds
- 2 cups coconut cream
- 1 teaspoon of cocoa powder
- 1 teaspoon vanilla extract
- 1 tablespoon Erythritol

Directions:

1. Pour the coconut cream in the air fryer.
2. Add cocoa powder, vanilla extract, and Erythritol. Stir the liquid until smooth.
3. Then cook it at 350F for 10 minutes.
4. Add chia seeds, carefully mix the dessert, and leave it to rest for 40 minutes.

Nutrition:
calories 442,
fat 42.6,
fiber 8.6,
carbs 15.3,
protein 6.1

Pumpkin Spices Muffins

Preparation time: 15 minutes
Cooking time: 10 minutes
Servings: 6
Ingredients:

- 1 cup coconut flour
- 1 tablespoon pumpkin spices
- ½ teaspoon baking powder
- 2 eggs, beaten
- 2 tablespoons coconut oil
- 2 tablespoons Erythritol

- 1 tablespoon coconut cream

Directions:

1. Mix all ingredients in the mixing bowl.
2. When the batter is smooth, pour it in the muffin molds and transfer in the air fryer basket.
3. Cook the muffins at 365F for 10 minutes.

Nutrition:
calories 149,
fat 8.7,
fiber 8.2,
carbs 14.4,
protein 4.6

Egg Custard

Preparation Time: 5 minutes
Cooking time: 30 minutes
Servings: 6
Ingredients:

- 6 eggs, beaten
- 2 cups heavy cream
- ½ cup Erythritol
- 1 teaspoon vanilla extract

Directions:

1. Whisk all ingredients until smooth and pour in the air fryer basket.
2. Cook the custard at 345F for 30 minutes.
3. Then cool it well.

Nutrition:
calories 203,
fat 19.2,
fiber 0
carbs 1.6,
protein 6.4

CHAPTER 11:

September

Lunch

Beef with Broccoli
Preparation time: 10 minutes
Cooking time: 13 minutes
Servings: 4
Ingredients:

- 6 oz. broccoli
- 10 oz. beef brisket
- 4 oz chive stems
- 1 teaspoon paprika
- 1/3 cup water
- 1 teaspoon olive oil
- 1 teaspoon butter
- 1 tablespoon flax seeds
- ½ teaspoon chili flakes

Directions:

1. Cut the beef brisket into medium pieces.
2. Coat the beef pieces with the paprika and chili flakes.
3. Combine using your hands.
4. Preheat the air fryer to 360 F.
5. Grease the air fryer basket tray with the olive oil.
6. Put the beef pieces in the air fryer basket tray and cook the meat for 7 minutes.
7. Stir once during the cooking.
8. Meanwhile, separate the broccoli into the florets.
9. Add the broccoli florets in the air fryer basket tray.
10. Sprinkle the ingredients with the flax seeds and butter.
11. Add water.
12. Dice the chives and add them in the air fryer basket tray.
13. Stir gently using the wooden spatula.
14. Cook the dish at 265 F for 6 minutes more.
15. When the broccoli is tender the dish is cooked.

Nutrition:
calories 187,
fat 7.3,
fiber 2.4,
carbs 6.2,
protein 23.4

Chicken Lasagna & Parmesan Eggplants
Preparation time: 21 minutes
Cooking time: 17 minutes
Servings: 10
Ingredients:

- 6 oz Cheddar cheese, shredded
- 7 oz Parmesan cheese, shredded

- 2 eggplants
- 1-pound ground chicken
- 1 teaspoon paprika
- 1 teaspoon salt
- ½ teaspoon cayenne pepper
- ½ cup heavy cream
- 2 teaspoon butter
- 4 oz chive stems, diced

Directions:
1. Take the air fryer basket tray and grease it with the butter.
2. Peel the eggplants and slice them.
3. Separate the sliced eggplants into 3 pieces.
4. Combine the ground chicken with the paprika, salt, cayenne pepper, and diced chives.
5. Combine well.
6. Separate the ground chicken mixture into 2 parts.
7. Make the first layer using the sliced eggplant in the air fryer basket tray.
8. Then make a second layer using the ground chicken mixture.
9. Sprinkle the chicken layer with half of the shredded Cheddar cheese,
10. Then cover the cheese with the second part of the sliced eggplant.
11. Make a layer of the ground chicken and all shredded Cheddar cheese,
12. Cover the cheese layer with the last part of the sliced eggplant.
13. Sprinkle the eggplants with shredded Parmesan cheese.
14. Pour the heavy cream and add butter.
15. Preheat the air fryer to 365 F.
16. Cook the lasagna for 17 minutes.

Nutrition:
calories 291,
fat 17.6,
fiber 4.6,
carbs 7.8,
protein 27.4

Garlic Beef Mash
Preparation time: 10 minutes
Cooking time: 15 minutes
Servings: 4
Ingredients:
- 1-pound ground beef
- 3 oz chive stems
- 1 teaspoon garlic, sliced
- 1 teaspoon ground white pepper
- ¼ cup cream
- 1 teaspoon olive oil
- 2 green peppers
- 1 teaspoon dried dill
- 1 teaspoon cayenne pepper
- 2 teaspoon chicken stock

Directions:
1. Dice the chive stems.
2. Combine the chives with the sliced garlic.
3. Combine the mixture carefully with a teaspoon.
4. Sprinkle the ground beef with the ground white pepper.

5. Add dried dill and cayenne pepper.
6. Grease the air fryer basket tray with the olive oil.
7. Preheat the air fryer to 365 F.
8. Put the spiced ground beef in the air fryer basket tray.
9. Cook the beef mixture for 3 minutes.
10. Stir it carefully.
11. Add the chives mixture and chicken stock.
12. Mix it gently and cook at the same temperature for 2 minutes more.
13. Meanwhile, chop the green peppers into the small pieces.
14. Add the chopped green peppers in the air fryer.
15. Add the cream and stir it until well combined.
16. Cook the ground beef mixture for 10 minutes more.
17. Mix the ground beef mixture with a hand blender.
18. Serve hot.

Nutrition:
calories 258, fat 9.3,
fiber 1.9,
carbs 6.8,
protein 35.5

Pork Meatballs Stuffed with Cheddar Cheese

Preparation time: 15 minutes
Cooking time: 8 minutes
Servings: 6
Ingredients:

- 1-pound ground pork
- 5 oz. Cheddar cheese
- 1 tablespoon dried oregano
- 1 large egg
- ½ teaspoon salt
- 1 teaspoon paprika
- 1 tablespoon butter
- ½ teaspoon nutmeg
- 1 teaspoon minced garlic
- ½ teaspoon ground ginger

Directions:

1. Crack the egg into a bowl and whisk it.
2. Add salt, paprika, nutmeg, and ground ginger to the bowl.
3. Stir gently and add the ground pork.
4. Add dried oregano and minced garlic.
5. Mix well using a spoon until well combined and make 6 medium balls.
6. Cut the Cheddar cheese into 6 medium cubes.
7. Fill the pork meatballs with the cheese cubes.
8. Preheat the air fryer to 365 F.
9. Toss the butter in the air fryer basket tray and melt it.
10. Add the pork meatballs and cook them for 8 minutes, stirring halfway through.

Nutrition:
calories 295,
fat 20.6,
fiber 0,
carbs 3,
protein 23

Chicken Liver Burgers

Preparation time: 15 minutes
Cooking time: 10 minutes
Servings: 7
Ingredients:

- ½ teaspoon turmeric
- ½ teaspoon ground coriander
- 1 teaspoon ground thyme
- ½ teaspoon salt
- 2 teaspoon butter
- 1 tablespoon almond flour
- 1 tablespoon coconut flour
- 1 teaspoon chili flakes
- 1-pound chicken liver
- 1 egg

Directions:

1. Grind the chicken liver.
2. Put the ground chicken in a mixing bowl.
3. Crack the egg in a separate bowl and whisk it.
4. Add the turmeric, ground coriander, ground thyme, and salt in the whisked egg mixture.
5. Add the whisked egg mixture to the ground liver.
6. Add the coconut flour and almond flour.
7. Mix with a spoon. You should get a non-sticky liver mixture. Add more almond flour if desired.
8. Preheat the air fryer to 360 F.
9. Then melt the butter and grease the air fryer basket tray with the melted butter.
10. Make medium liver burgers and put them in the Prepared air fryer basket tray.
11. Cook the burgers for 5 minutes on each side. The burger should be a little bit crunchy.
12. When the liver burgers are cooked – let them chill a little before serving.

Nutrition:
calories 155,
fat 8.1,
fiber 0.9,
carbs 2.4,
protein 17.7

Paprika Turkey Rolls

Preparation time: 10 minutes
Cooking time: 12 minutes
Servings: 4
Ingredients:

- 1-pound turkey fillet
- 2 tablespoon garlic clove, sliced
- 1 teaspoon apple cider vinegar
- 3 oz chive stems
- ½ teaspoon salt
- 1 teaspoon paprika
- 1 teaspoon dried dill
- 1 tablespoon chives powder
- 4 teaspoon butter

Directions:

1. Cut the turkey fillet into 4 parts.
2. Then tenderize each turkey fillet gently.
3. Coat the turkey fillets with the apple cider vinegar, salt, paprika, and dried dill.

4. Chop the chives and combine it with the sliced garlic clove.
5. Add the chives powder and butter.
6. Mix the mixture until well combined.
7. Place the churned garlic mixture in the center of each turkey fillet.
8. Roll the fillets and secure with the toothpicks.
9. Preheat the air fryer to 360 F.
10. Put the turkey rolls in the air fryer basket tray and cook the dish for 12 minutes.
11. Turn the rolls over midway through cooking.
12. Transfer the cooked juicy turkey rolls on the plate and serve them hot.

Nutrition:
calories 155,
fat 4.5,
fiber 0.6,
carbs 3.2,
protein 24.2

Spinach & Cabbage Chicken Stew
Preparation time: 15 minutes
Cooking time: 12 minutes
Servings: 6
Ingredients:
- 8 oz. chicken breast
- 3 oz chive stems
- ½ cup spinach
- 2 cups chicken stock
- 5 oz. white cabbage
- 6 oz. cauliflower
- 1/3 cup heavy cream
- 1 teaspoon salt
- 1 green pepper
- 1 teaspoon paprika
- 1 teaspoon cayenne pepper
- 1 teaspoon butter
- 1 teaspoon ground cilantro

Directions:
1. Cut the chicken breast into the large cubes.
2. Coat the chicken cubes with the salt, paprika, cayenne pepper, and ground cilantro.
3. Preheat the air fryer to 365 F.
4. Put the butter in the air fryer basket tray and melt it.
5. Add the chicken cubes and cook them for 4 minutes.
6. Meanwhile, chop the spinach and dice the chives.
7. Shred the cabbage and cut the cauliflower into the small florets.
8. Chop the green pepper.
9. Add all the Prepared ingredients in the air fryer basket tray.
10. Pour the heavy cream and chicken stock.
11. Set the air fryer to 360 F and cook the stew for 8 minutes more.
12. When the stew is cooked – stir it gently with a spatula.
13. Serve the cooked chicken stew immediately.

Nutrition:
calories 102, fat 4.5,
fiber 2.3,
carbs 6.4,
protein 9.8

Cheddar Chicken Pizza

Preparation time: 15 minutes
Cooking time: 12 minutes
Servings: 6
Ingredients:

- 10 oz. ground chicken
- 1 teaspoon minced garlic
- 1 teaspoon almond flour
- ½ teaspoon salt
- 1 teaspoon ground black pepper
- 1 large egg
- 6 oz. Cheddar cheese, shredded
- ½ teaspoon dried dill

Directions:

1. Put the ground chicken in a bowl.
2. Coat it with the minced garlic, almond flour, salt, ground black pepper, and dried dill.
3. Crack the egg into the ground chicken mixture and mix with a spoon.
4. Combine to get a smooth texture.
5. Preheat the air fryer to 380 F.
6. Cover the air fryer pizza tray with the parchment.
7. Place the ground chicken mixture in the air fryer pizza tray and make the shape of a pizza crust.
8. Cook the chicken pizza crust for 8 minutes.
9. Remove the chicken pizza crust from the air fryer and sprinkle it with the shredded cheese generously.
10. Cook the pizza for 4 minutes more at 365 F.

Nutrition:
calories 244,
fat 16.1,
fiber 0.6,
carbs 1.9,
protein 22.9

Dinner

Chimichurri Skirt Steak

Basic Recipe
Preparation Time: 10 minutes
Cooking Time: 8 minutes
Servings: 2
Ingredients:

- 2 x 8 oz. skirt steak
- 1 cup finely chopped parsley
- ¼ cup finely chopped mint
- 2 tbsp. fresh oregano (washed & finely chopped)
- 3 finely chopped cloves of garlic
- 1 tsp. red pepper flakes (crushed)
- 1 tbsp. ground cumin
- 1 tsp. cayenne pepper
- 2 tsp. smoked paprika
- 1 tsp. salt
- ¼ tsp. pepper
- ¾ cup oil
- 3 tbsp. red wine vinegar

Directions:

1. Throw all the ingredients in a bowl (besides the steak) and mix well.
2. Put ¼ cup of the mixture in a plastic baggie with the steak and leave in the fridge overnight (2–24hrs).

3. Leave the bag out at room temperature for at least 30 min before popping into the air fryer. Preheat for a minute or two to 390° F before cooking until med–rare (8–10 min). Pour into the Oven rack/basket. Place the Rack on the middle-shelf of the Air Fryer Oven. Set temperature to 390°F, and set time to 10 minutes

4. Put 2 Tbsp. of the chimichurri mix on top of each steak before serving.

Nutrition:
Calories 308.6 Cal
Fat 22.6 g
Carbs 3 g
Protein 23.7 g

Country Fried Steak
Basic Recipe
Preparation Time: 5 minutes
Cooking Time: 12 minutes
Servings: 2
Ingredients:

- 1 tsp. pepper
- 2 C. almond milk
- 2 tbsp. almond flour
- 6 ounces ground sausage meat
- 1 tsp. pepper
- 1 tsp. salt
- 1 tsp. garlic powder
- 1 tsp. onion powder
- 1 C. panko breadcrumbs
- 1 C. almond flour
- 3 beaten eggs
- 6 ounces sirloin steak, pounded till thin

Directions:

1. Season panko breadcrumbs with spices
2. Dredge steak in flour, then egg, and then seasoned panko mixture.
3. Place into air fryer basket.
4. Set temperature to 370°F, and set time to 12 minutes
5. To make sausage gravy, cook sausage and Dry outof fat, but reserve 2 tablespoons.
6. Add flour to sausage and mix until incorporated. Gradually mix in milk over medium to high heat till it becomes thick.
7. Season mixture with pepper and cook 3 minutes longer.
8. Serve steak topped with gravy and enjoy.

Nutrition:
Calories 395 Cal
Fat 11 g
Carbs 0 g
Protein 39 g

Creamy Burger
Intermediate Recipe
Preparation Time: 5 minutes
Cooking Time: 55 minutes
Servings: 3
Ingredients:

- Salt to taste
- Freshly ground pepper, to taste
- 1/2 (10.75 ounce) can condensed cream of mushroom soup
- 1/2-pound lean ground beef
- 1/2 cup shredded Cheddar cheese
- 1/4 cup chopped onion
- 1/4 cup and 2 tablespoons milk

Directions:

1. Lightly grease baking pan of air fryer with cooking spray. Add ground beef. For 10 minutes, cook on 360°F
2. Stir and crumble halfway through cooking time.
3. Meanwhile, in a bowl, whisk well pepper, salt, milk, onion, and mushroom soup. Mix well.
4. Dry out fat off ground beef and transfer beef to a plate.
5. Cover pan with foil.
6. Cook for 30 minutes Remove foil and cook for another 15 minutes.
7. Serve and enjoy.

Nutrition:
Calories 399 Cal
Fat 26.9 g
Carbs 0 g
Protein 22.1 g

Beefy 'n Cheesy Spanish Cauliflower Rice Casserole

Intermediate Recipe
Preparation Time: 10 minutes
Cooking Time: 50 minutes
Servings: 3
Ingredients:

- 2 tablespoons chopped green bell pepper
- 1 tablespoon chopped fresh cilantro
- 1/2-pound lean ground beef
- 1/2 cup water
- 1/2 teaspoon salt
- 1/2 teaspoon brown sugar
- 1/2 pinch ground black pepper
- 1/3 cup cooked cauliflower rice
- 1/4 cup finely chopped onion
- 1/4 cup chili sauce
- 1/4 teaspoon ground cumin
- 1/4 teaspoon Worcestershire sauce
- 1/4 cup shredded Cheddar cheese

Directions:

1. Lightly grease baking pan of air fryer with cooking spray. Add ground beef.
2. For 10 minutes, cook on 360°F Halfway through cooking time, stir and crumble beef. Discard excess fat,
3. Stir in pepper, Worcestershire sauce, cumin, brown sugar, salt, chili sauce, cauliflower rice, water, green bell pepper, and onion. Mix well. Cover pan with foil and cook for 25 minutes. Stirring occasionally
4. Give it one last good stir, press down firmly and sprinkle cheese on top.
5. Cook uncovered for 15 minutes at 390°F until tops are lightly browned.
6. Serve and enjoy with chopped cilantro.

Nutrition:
Calories 346 CalFat 19.1 g
Carbs 0 g Protein 18.5 g

Warming Winter Beef with Celery

Basic Recipe
Preparation Time: 5 minutes
Cooking Time: 12 minutes
Servings: 4
Ingredients:

- 9 ounces tender beef, chopped
- 1/2 cup leeks, chopped
- 1/2 cup celery stalks, chopped

- 2 cloves garlic, smashed
- 2 tablespoons red cooking wine
- 3/4 cup cream of celery soup
- 2 sprigs rosemary, chopped
- 1/4 teaspoon smoked paprika
- 3/4 teaspoons salt
- 1/4 teaspoon black pepper, or to taste

Directions:
1. Add the beef, lccks, celery, and garlic to the baking dish; cook for about 5 minutes at 390 degrees F.
2. Once the meat is starting to tender, pour in the wine and soup. Season with rosemary, smoked paprika, salt, and black pepper
3. Now, cook an additional 7 minutes

Nutrition:
Calories 364 Cal Fat 9 g
Carbs 39 g Protein 32 g

Beef & veggie Spring Rolls

Basic Recipe
Preparation Time: 5 minutes
Cooking Time: 12 minutes
Servings: 10
Ingredients:
- 2-ounce Asian noodles
- 1 tablespoon sesame oil
- 7-ounce ground beef
- 1 small onion, chopped
- 3 garlic cloves, crushed
- 1 cup fresh mixed vegetables
- 1 teaspoon soy sauce
- 1 packet spring roll skins
- 2 tablespoons water
- Olive oil, as required

Directions:
1. Soak the noodles in warm water till soft.
2. Dry out and cut into small lengths. In a pan heat the oil and add the onion and garlic and sauté for about 4-5 minutes
3. Add beef and cook for about 4-5 minutes
4. Add vegetables and cook for about 5-7 minutes or till cooked through.
5. Stir in soy sauce and remove from the heat.
6. Immediately, stir in the noodles and keep aside till all the juices have been absorbed.
7. Preheat the Air Fryer Oven to 350 degrees F.
8. Place the spring rolls skin onto a smooth surface.
9. Add a line of the filling diagonally across.
10. Fold the top point over the filling and then fold in both sides.
11. On the final point, brush it with water before rolling to seal.
12. Brush the spring rolls with oil.
13. Arrange the rolls in batches in the air fryer and Cook for about 8 minutes
14. Repeat with remaining rolls. Now, place spring rolls onto a baking sheet.
15. Bake it for about 6 minutes per side.

Nutrition:
Calories 364 Cal
Fat 9 g
Carbs 39 g
Protein 32 g

Meat

Pork And Fruit Kebabs

Preparation Time: 15 minutes
Cooking Time: 9-12 minutes
Servings: 4
Ingredients:

- ⅓ cup apricot jam
- 2 tablespoons freshly squeezed lemon juice
- 2 teaspoons olive oil
- ½ teaspoon dried tarragon
- 1 (1-pound) pork tenderloin, cut into 1-inch cubes
- 4 plums, pitted and quartered (see Tip)
- 4 small apricots, pitted and halved (see Tip)

Directions:

1. In a large bowl, mix the jam, lemon juice, olive oil, and tarragon.
2. Add the pork and stir to coat. Let stand for 10 minutes at room temperature.
3. Alternating the items, thread the pork, plums, and -apricots onto 4 metal skewers that fit into the air fryer. Brush with any remaining jam mixture. Discard any remaining marinade.
4. Grill the kebabs in the air fryer for 9 to 12 minutes, or until the pork reaches 145°F on a meat thermometer and the fruit is tender. Serve immediately.

Nutrition:
Calories: 256
Fat; 5g
Saturated Fat; 1g
Protein: 24g
 Carbohydrates: 30g
Sodium: 60mg
Fiber: 2g
Sugar: 22g

Steak And Vegetable Kebabs

Preparation Time: 15 minutes
Cooking Time: 5 to 7 minutes
Servings: 4
Ingredients:

- 2 tablespoons balsamic vinegar
- 2 teaspoons olive oil
- ½ teaspoon dried marjoram
- ⅛ teaspoon freshly ground black pepper
- ¾ pound round steak, cut into 1-inch pieces
- 1 red bell pepper, sliced
- 16 button mushrooms

Directions:

1. In a medium bowl, stir together the balsamic vinegar, olive oil, marjoram, and black pepper.
2. Add the steak and stir to coat. Let stand for 10 minutes at room temperature.
3. Alternating items, thread the beef, red bell pepper, mushrooms, onto 8 bamboo or metal skewers that fit in the air fryer.
4. Grill in the air fryer for 5 to 7 minutes, or until the beef is browned and reaches at least 145°F on a meat thermo-meter. Serve immediately.

Nutrition:
Calories: 194
Fat: 6g
 Saturated Fat: 2g
Protein: 31g

Carbohydrates: 7g
Sodium: 53mg
Fiber: 2g
Sugar: 2g

Spicy Grilled Steak

Preparation Time: 7 minutes
Cooking Time: 6 to 9 minutes
Servings: 4
Ingredients:

- 2 tablespoons low-sodium salsa
- 1 tablespoon minced chipotle pepper
- 1 tablespoon apple cider vinegar
- 1 teaspoon ground cumin
- ⅛ teaspoon freshly ground black pepper
- ⅛ teaspoon red pepper flakes
- ¾ pound sirloin tip steak, cut into 4 pieces and gently pounded to about ⅓ inch thick

Directions:

1. In a small bowl, thoroughly mix the salsa, chipotle pepper, cider vinegar, cumin, black pepper, and red pepper flakes. Rub this mixture into both sides of each steak piece. Let stand for 15 minutes at room temperature.
2. Grill the steaks in the air fryer, two at a time, for 6 to 9 minutes, or until they reach at least 145°F on a meat thermometer.
3. Remove the steaks to a clean plate and cover with aluminum foil to keep warm. Repeat with the remaining steaks.
4. Slice the steaks thinly against the grain and serve.

Nutrition:
Calories: 160
Fat: 6g

Saturated Fat: 3g
Protein: 24g
Carbohydrates: 1g
Sodium: 87mg
Fiber: 0g
Sugar: 0g

Fish

Easy Tuna Patties

Preparation Time: 10 minutes
Cooking Time: 10 minutes
Servings: 5
Ingredients:

- 15 oz can albacore tuna, drained
- 1/2 teaspoon dried mix herbs
- 1/2 teaspoon garlic powder
- 3 tablespoon onion, minced
- 1 celery stalk, chopped
- 3 tablespoon parmesan cheese, grated
- 1/2 cup almond flour
- 1 tablespoon lemon juice
- 2 large eggs, lightly beaten

Directions:

1. Add all ingredients into the mixing bowl and mix until well combined.
2. Make the equal shape of patties from the mixture.
3. Place the cooking tray in the air fryer basket. Line air fryer basket with parchment paper.
4. Select Air Fry mode.
5. Set time to 10 minutes and temperature 360 F then press START.
6. The air fryer display will prompt you to ADD FOOD once the temperature is reached then place patties in the air fryer basket.
7. Turn patties halfway through.
8. Serve and enjoy.

Nutrition:
Calories 138
Fat 4.9 g
Carbohydrates 2.2 g
Sugar 0.7 g
Protein 21.2 g
Cholesterol 107 mg

Old Bay Shrimp

Preparation Time: 10 minutes
Cooking Time: 10 minutes
Servings: 4
Ingredients:

- 1 lb shrimp, peeled & deveined
- 1 tablespoon old bay seasoning
- 1/2 tablespoon garlic, minced
- 1/2 tablespoon lemon juice
- 1/2 tablespoon olive oil

Directions:

1. Add shrimp and remaining ingredients into the mixing bowl and toss well.
2. Place the cooking tray in the air fryer basket.
3. Select Air Fry mode.
4. Set time to 10 minutes and temperature 390 F then press START.
5. The air fryer display will prompt you to ADD FOOD once the temperature is reached then add shrimp in the air fryer basket.
6. Serve and enjoy.

Nutrition:
Calories 152
Fat 3.7 g
Carbohydrates 2.1 g
Sugar 0.1 g
Protein 25.9 g
Cholesterol 239 mg

Baked Mahi Mahi

Preparation Time: 10 minutes
Cooking Time: 30 minutes
Servings: 4
Ingredients:

- 4 Mahi Mahi fillets
- 1 teaspoon onion powder
- 1 teaspoon garlic powder
- 1 teaspoon turmeric
- 1 tablespoon dried basil
- 1 teaspoon pepper
- 1 teaspoon salt

Directions:

1. In a small bowl, mix together onion powder, garlic powder,

turmeric, basil, pepper, and salt.

2. Season fish fillets with spice mixture.
3. Place the cooking tray in the air fryer basket. Line air fryer basket with parchment paper.
4. Select Bake mode.
5. Set time to 30 minutes and temperature 350 F then press START.
6. The air fryer display will prompt you to ADD FOOD once the temperature is reached then place the fish fillet in the air fryer basket.
7. Serve and enjoy.

Nutrition:
Calories 108
Fat 1.1 g
Carbohydrates 2.7 g
Sugar 0.4 g
Protein 21.3 g
Cholesterol 80 mg

Vegetable

Cheese Broccoli Stuffed Pepper
Preparation Time: 10 minutes
Cooking Time: 25 minutes
Servings: 4
Ingredients:

- 4 eggs
- 2.5 oz cheddar cheese, grated
- 2 medium bell peppers, cut in half and deseeded
- 2 tablespoon olive oil
- 1/4 cup baby broccoli florets
- 1 teaspoon dried sage
- 7 oz unsweetened almond milk
- Pepper
- Salt

Directions:

1. In a bowl, whisk together eggs, milk, broccoli, sage, pepper, and salt.
2. Add olive oil to the baking dish.
3. Place bell pepper halves in the baking dish.
4. Pour egg mixture into the bell pepper halves.
5. Sprinkle cheese on top of bell pepper.
6. Select Bake mode.
7. Set time to 25 minutes and temperature 390 F then press START.
8. The air fryer display will prompt you to ADD FOOD once the temperature is reached then place the baking dish in the air fryer basket.
9. Serve and enjoy.

Nutrition:
Calories 226
Fat 18.1 g
Carbohydrates 6.3 g
Sugar 3.9 g
Protein 10.9 g
Cholesterol 182 mg

Beans with Mushrooms
Preparation Time: 10 minutes
Cooking Time: 25 minutes
Servings: 4
Ingredients:

- 2 cups mushrooms, sliced
- 2 teaspoon garlic, minced

- 2 cups green beans, clean and cut into pieces
- 1/4 cup olive oil
- 1 teaspoon black pepper
- 1 teaspoon sea salt

Directions:

1. In a bowl, mix together olive oil, pepper, garlic, and salt.
2. Pour olive oil mixture over green beans and mushrooms and stir to coat.
3. Spread green beans and mushroom mixture into the baking dish.
4. Select Bake mode.
5. Set time to 25 minutes and temperature 400 F then press START.
6. The air fryer display will prompt you to ADD FOOD once the temperature is reached then place the baking dish in the air fryer basket.
7. Serve and enjoy.

Nutrition:
Calories 136
Fat 12.8 g
Carbohydrates 5.9 g
Sugar 1.4 g
Protein 2.3 g
Cholesterol 0 mg

Basil Pesto Spaghetti Squash

Preparation Time: 10 minutes

Cooking Time: 10 minutes

Serve: 4

Ingredients:

- 2 cups spaghetti squash, cooked and drained
- 4 oz mozzarella cheese, cubed
- 1/4 cup basil pesto
- 1/2 cup ricotta cheese
- 1 tbsp olive oil
- Pepper
- Salt

Directions:

1. In a bowl, combine together olive oil and squash. Season with pepper and salt.
2. Spread squash mixture in greased baking dish.
3. Spread mozzarella cheese and ricotta cheese on top.
4. Select BAKE mode, then set the temperature to 375 F and the time to 10 minutes, then press start.
5. When the display shows Add Food then place the baking dish in the vortex plus air fryer oven.
6. Drizzle with basil pesto and serve.

Nutrition:

Calories 169

Fat 11.3 g

Carbohydrates 6.1 g

Sugar 0.1 g

Protein 11.9 g

Cholesterol 25 mg

Carbohydrates 10.4 g
Sugar 4.8 g
Protein 7 g
Cholesterol 10 mg

Parmesan Eggplant Zucchini

Preparation Time: 10 minutes
Cooking Time: 35 minutes
Servings: 6
Ingredients:

- 1 medium eggplant, sliced
- 3 medium zucchini, sliced
- 3 oz Parmesan cheese, grated
- 1 tablespoon olive oil
- 4 garlic cloves, minced
- 4 tablespoon parsley, chopped
- 4 tablespoon basil, chopped
- 1/4 teaspoon pepper
- 1/4 teaspoon salt

Directions:

1. In a mixing bowl, add chopped eggplant, zucchini, olive oil, garlic, cheese, basil, pepper, and salt toss well until combined.
2. Transfer the eggplant mixture into the baking dish.
3. Select Bake mode.
4. Set time to 35 minutes and temperature 350 F then press START.
5. The air fryer display will prompt you to ADD FOOD once the temperature is reached then place the baking dish in the air fryer basket.
6. Serve and enjoy.

Nutrition:
Calories 110
Fat 5.8 g

Snacks

Creamy Broccoli Crisps

Preparation time: 15 minutes
Cooking time: 13 minutes
Servings: 6
Ingredients:

- 3 tablespoon heavy cream
- 1 tablespoon almond flour
- ½ teaspoon salt
- ½ teaspoon turmeric
- 1 teaspoon ground black pepper
- 1-pound broccoli

Directions:

1. Wash the broccoli and separate it into small florets.
2. Then combine the almond flour, salt, turmeric, and ground black pepper in a shallow spice bowl.
3. Shake to combine well.
4. Sprinkle the florets with the spice mixture.
5. Stir carefully.
6. Drizzle the broccoli florets with the heavy cream and mix well.
7. Sprinkle the broccoli florets with the remaining spices one more time.
8. Preheat the air fryer to 360 F.

9. Put the Prepared broccoli florets in the air fryer rack.

10.Cook the broccoli florets for 10 minutes.

11.Shake the broccoli carefully.

12.Cook the broccoli crisps for 3 minutes more.

13.Let the cooked broccoli crisps cool before serving.

Nutrition:

calories 80,

fat 5.4,

fiber 2.6,

carbs 6.6,

protein 3.3

Spicy Kale Chips

Preparation time: 10 minutes

Cooking time: 8 minutes

Servings: 14

Ingredients:

- 1-pound kale
- 1 teaspoon salt
- 1 teaspoon chili pepper
- 2 teaspoon olive oil

Directions:

1. Wash the kale and dry well.

2. Tear the kale roughly.

3. Preheat the air fryer to 370 F.

4. Sprinkle the kale with salt, chili pepper, and olive oil.

5. Mix well.

6. Place the kale on the air fryer rack and cook for 5 minutes.

7. Shake the kale and cook it for 3 minutes more.

8. Chill the chips and keep them in a dry place.

Nutrition:

calories 22, fat 0.7,

fiber 0.5, carbs 3.4,

protein 1

Paprika Kohlrabi Chips

Preparation time: 7 minutes

Cooking time: 20 minutes

Servings: 10

Ingredients:

- 1-pound kohlrabi
- 1 teaspoon salt
- 1 tablespoon sesame oil
- 1 teaspoon smoked paprika

Directions:

1. Peel the kohlrabi.

2. Slice it into thin pieces.

3. Sprinkle the kohlrabi slices with salt, smoked paprika, and sesame oil.

4. Shake the mixture.

5. Preheat the air fryer to 320 F.

6. Put the kohlrabi slices in the air fryer rack and cook for 20 minutes.

7. Stir during cooking.

8. Cool before serving.

Nutrition:

calories 25,

fat 1.4,

fiber 1.7,

carbs 2.9,

protein 0.8

Kohlrabi French Fries

Preparation time: 10 minutes

Cooking time: 20 minutes

Servings: 8

Ingredients:

- 1 egg
- 2 tablespoon almond flour
- ½ teaspoon salt
- 1 teaspoon ground black pepper
- 1 teaspoon thyme
- 1 tablespoon olive oil
- 14 oz. kohlrabi

Directions:

1. Crack the egg into a bowl and whisk.
2. Sprinkle the whisked egg with the salt, ground black pepper, and thyme.
3. Whisk for 1 minute.
4. Peel the kohlrabi and cut it into French fries.
5. Put the kohlrabi pieces in the whisked egg mixture.
6. Coat the kohlrabi in the almond flour.
7. Preheat the air fryer to 360 F.
8. Coat the kohlrabi with olive oil and put in the air fryer.
9. Cook for 20 minutes.
10. Stir frequently.
11. Allow to cool before serving.

Nutrition:
calories 77,
fat 5.9,
fiber 2.7,
carbs 4.9,
protein 3.1

Dessert

Ricotta Muffins

Preparation time: 15 minutes
Cooking time: 11 minutes
Servings: 4
Ingredients:

- 4 teaspoons ricotta cheese
- 1 egg, beaten
- ½ teaspoon baking powder
- 1 teaspoon vanilla extract
- 8 teaspoons coconut flour
- 3 tablespoons coconut cream
- 2 teaspoons Erythritol
- Cooking spray

Directions:

1. Spray the muffin molds with cooking spray.
2. Then mix all ingredients in the mixing bowl.
3. When you get a smooth batter, pour it in the muffin molds and place in the air fryer basket.
4. Cook the muffins at 365F for 11 minutes.

Nutrition:
calories 72,
fat 4.7,
fiber 2.3,
carbs 4.7,
protein 2.9

Keto Sponge

Preparation time: 10 minutes
Cooking time: 30 minutes
Servings: 6
Ingredients:

- 2 cups coconut flour
- 5 eggs, beaten

- ½ cup Erythritol
- 1 teaspoon baking powder
- 1 teaspoon vanilla extract
- Cooking spray

Directions:

1. Whisk the coconut flour with eggs, Erythritol, baking powder, and vanilla extract.
2. Spray the baking pan with cooking spray and pour the coconut flour mixture inside.
3. Put the pan in the air fryer basket and cook at 355F for 30 minutes.

Nutrition:
calories 75,
fat 4.3,
fiber 1.7,
carbs 3.4,
protein 5.3

Baked Cantaloupe

Preparation Time: 10 minutes
Cooking time: 10 minutes
Servings: 2
Ingredients:

- 1 cup cantaloupe, chopped
- 1 teaspoon vanilla extract
- 1 tablespoon Erythritol
- 1 teaspoon olive oil

Directions:

1. Put the cantaloupe in the air fryer basket and sprinkle with vanilla extract, Erythritol, and olive oil.
2. Cook the dessert at 375F for 10 minutes.

Nutrition:
calories 53,
fat 2.5,
fiber 0.7,
carbs 6.6,
protein 0.7

Rhubarb Pie

Preparation time: 15 minutes
Cooking time: 20 minutes
Servings: 6
Ingredients:

- 4 oz rhubarb, chopped
- ¼ cup coconut cream
- 1 teaspoon vanilla extract
- ¼ cup Erythritol
- 1 cup coconut flour
- 1 egg, beaten
- 4 tablespoons coconut oil, softened

Directions:

1. Mix coconut cream with vanilla extract, Erythritol, coconut flour, egg, and coconut oil.
2. When the mixture is smooth, add rhubarb and stir gently.
3. Pour the mixture in the air fryer and cook the pie at 375F for 20 minutes.
4. Cool the cooked pie and cut into servings.

Nutrition:
calories 198,
fat 14.2,
fiber 8.6,
carbs 14.9,
protein 4

Butter Cookies

Preparation time: 15 minutes
Cooking time: 10 minutes
Servings: 5
Ingredients:

- 4 tablespoons butter, softened
- 4 teaspoons Splenda
- 1 egg, beaten
- 1 cup coconut flour

Directions:

1. In the mixing bowl, mix butter, Splenda, egg, and coconut flour.
2. Knead the dough and make the balls (cookies).
3. Put them in the air fryer and cook at 365F for 10 minutes.

Nutrition:
calories 206, fat 12.5,
fiber 9.6, carbs 19.3,
protein 4.4

Mascarpone Brownies

Preparation Time: 10 minutes
Cooking time: 25 minutes
Servings: 6
Ingredients:

- 6 tablespoons mascarpone
- 3 eggs, beaten
- 2 tablespoons cocoa powder
- 3 tablespoons butter, softened
- 1 cup almond flour
- ¼ teaspoon baking soda
- ¼ cup coconut cream
- 3 tablespoons Erythritol

Directions:

1. Mix all ingredients in the mixing bowl until smooth.
2. Then line the air fryer basket with baking paper and pour the brownie batter inside.
3. Cook the meal at 360F for 25 minutes.
4. Then cool the dessert little and cut into brownies.

Nutrition:
calories 248,
fat 21.5,
fiber 2.8,
carbs 6.2,
protein 9.1

Chia Balls

Preparation time: 15 minutes
Cooking time: 10 minutes
Servings: 4
Ingredients:

- 4 teaspoons chia seeds
- 1 tablespoon coconut oil, softened
- 1 tablespoon Erythritol
- ½ teaspoon vanilla extract
- 1 tablespoon almond flour
- 1 teaspoon almond flakes
- 1 egg, beaten
- Cooking spray

Directions:

1. Spray the air fryer basket with cooking spray.
2. Then mix all remaining ingredients in the mixing bowl and stir until homogenous.
3. Make the balls from the mixture and put in the air fryer in one layer.
4. Cook the chia balls at 365F for 10 minutes.

Nutrition:
calories 126,
fat 9.7,
fiber 5.1,
carbs 10.2,
protein 4.1

Coconut Cream Cups

Preparation Time: 5 minutes
Cooking time: 10 minutes
Servings: 2
Ingredients:

- 1 cup coconut cream
- 4 egg yolks
- 2 tablespoons Erythritol

- 1 tablespoon coconut flour
- 1 teaspoon vanilla extract

Directions:
1. Whisk the egg yolks with coconut cream and Erythritol.
2. Then add coconut flour and vanilla extract. Whisk the mixture until smooth.
3. Pour the mixture in the baking cups and put it in the air fryer basket.
4. Cook the cups at 390F for 10 minutes.

Nutrition:
calories 105,
fat 3.8,
fiber 4.1,
carbs 10.6,
protein 8.6

Cream Cheese Bombs

Preparation time: 10 minutes
Cooking time: 5 minutes

Servings: 2
Ingredients:
- 2 tablespoons cream cheese
- 4 tablespoons coconut flour
- 1 teaspoon vanilla extract
- 1 egg, beaten
- 1 tablespoon Erythritol
- 2 tablespoons coconut shred

Directions:
1. Mix cream cheese with coconut flour, vanilla extract, egg, Erythritol, and coconut shred.
2. Make the balls from the mixture and put in the air fryer basket.
3. Cook the cheese bombs at 390F for 5 minutes.

Nutrition:
calories 166,
fat 10.5,
fiber 6.7,
carbs 12,
protein 5.9

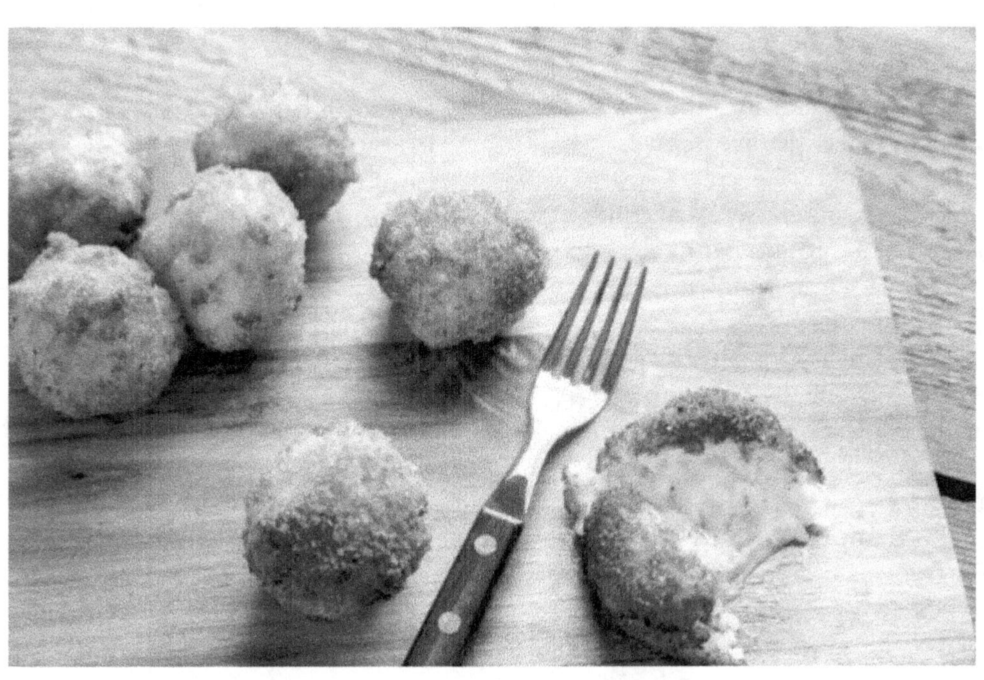

CHAPTER 12:

October

<u>Lunch</u>

Corn Chive Beef
Preparation time: 10 minutes
Cooking time: 19 minutes
Servings: 3
Ingredients:

- 3 oz chive stems
- 1 teaspoon black pepper
- ¼ teaspoon cayenne pepper
- 1 cup water
- 1-pound minced beef
- 1 teaspoon butter
- ½ teaspoon ground paprika

Directions:

1. Dice the chives finely.
2. Pour water into the pizza tray and place the diced chives.
3. Sprinkle the chives with the black pepper, cayenne pepper, and ground paprika.
4. Add water and mix the chives up carefully.
5. Preheat the air fryer to 400 F and put the tray into the air fryer basket.
6. Cook the chives for 4 minutes.
7. Remove the tray from the air fryer and add the minced garlic.
8. Combine the chives-meat mixture carefully and return it back in the air fryer.
9. Cook the beef mixture for 7 minutes at the same temperature.
10. Mix the meat mixture carefully with the help of a fork and cook for 8 minutes more.
11. Remove the cooked beef from the air fryer and mix it gently with a fork.
12. Transfer the cooked beef to serving plates.

Nutrition:
calories 310, fat 10.8,
fiber 1.2, carbs 4.2, protein 46.4

Pepper Beef Stew
Preparation time: 15 minutes
Cooking time: 23 minutes
Servings: 6
Ingredients:

- 10 oz. beef short ribs
- 1 cup chicken stock
- 1 garlic clove
- 3 oz chive stems
- 4 oz. green peas
- ¼ teaspoon salt
- 1 teaspoon turmeric
- 1 green pepper
- 2 teaspoon butter

- ½ teaspoon chili flakes
- 4 oz. kale

Directions:

1. Preheat the air fryer to 360 F.
2. Place the butter in the air fryer basket tray.
3. Add the beef short ribs.
4. Sprinkle the beef short ribs with the salt, turmeric, and chili flakes.
5. Cook the beef short ribs for 15 minutes.
6. Meanwhile, remove the seeds from the green pepper and chop it.
7. Chop the kale and dice the chives.
8. When the time is over – pour the chicken stock in the beef short ribs.
9. Add the chopped green pepper and diced chives.
10. After this, sprinkle the mixture with the green peas.
11. Peel the garlic clove and add it to the mixture too.
12. Mix it up using the wooden spatula.
13. Then chop the kale and add it to the stew mixture.
14. Stir the stew mixture one more time and cook it at 360 F for 8 minutes more.
15. When the stew is cooked – let it rest little.
16. Then mix the stew up and transfer to the serving plates.
17. Enjoy!

Nutrition:
calories 144, fat 5.8, fiber 1.9, carbs 7, protein 15.7

Garlic Chicken Curry

Preparation time: 10 minutes
Cooking time: 15 minutes
Servings: 4
Ingredients:

- 1 teaspoon olive oil
- 1-pound chicken breast, skinless, boneless
- 5 oz chive stems
- 2 teaspoon minced garlic
- 1 tablespoon apple cider vinegar
- 1 tablespoon lemongrass
- ½ cup coconut milk
- ½ cup chicken stock
- 2 tablespoon curry paste

Directions:

1. Cut the chicken breast into cubes,
2. Dice the chives.
3. Combine the chicken cubes and diced chives together in the air fryer basket tray.
4. Preheat the air fryer to 365 F.
5. Put the chicken mixture in the air fryer and cook it for 5 minutes.
6. Add the minced garlic, apple cider vinegar, lemongrass, coconut milk, chicken stock, and curry paste.
7. Combine the mixture using a wooden spatula.
8. Cook the chicken curry for 10 minutes more at the same temperature.
9. Stir before serving.

Nutrition:
calories 275, fat 15.7, fiber 1.3, carbs 7.2, protein 25.6

Thyme Shredded Beef

Preparation time: 15 minutes
Cooking time: 22 minutes
Servings: 8
Ingredients:

- 1 teaspoon thyme
- 1 teaspoon ground black pepper
- 1 teaspoon salt
- 1 teaspoon dried dill
- 1 teaspoon mustard
- 4 cup chicken stock
- 2-pound beef steak
- 1 garlic clove, peeled
- 3 tablespoon butter
- 1 bay leaf

Directions:

1. Preheat the air fryer to 360 F.
2. Meanwhile, combine the thyme, ground black pepper, salt, dried dill, and mustard in a small mixing bowl.
3. Sprinkle the beefsteak with the spice mixture on each side.
4. Massage the beefsteak using your fingertips to help the meat absorb the spices.
5. Pour the chicken stock in the air fryer.
6. Add the Prepared beef steak and bay leaf.
7. Cook the beefsteak for 20 minutes.
8. Strain the chicken stock and remove the beefsteak from the air fryer.
9. Shred the meat using 2 forks and return it back in the air fryer basket tray.
10. Add butter and cook the meat for 2 minutes at 365 F.
11. Mix the shredded meat carefully using a fork.
12. Transfer the dish to serving bowls.

Nutrition:
calories 265,
fat 14,
fiber 0.2,
carbs 1.2,
protein 32.4

Beef Strips with Zucchini Zoodles

Preparation time: 15 minutes
Cooking time: 13 minutes
Servings: 8
Ingredients:

- 1-pound beef brisket
- 1 teaspoon ground black pepper
- 1 teaspoon salt
- 1 zucchini
- 1 teaspoon olive oil
- 1 teaspoon Italian spices
- 4 tablespoon water

Directions:

1. Cut the beef brisket into strips.
2. Sprinkle the beef strips with the ground black pepper and salt.
3. Blend well until you get a smooth puree.
4. Grease the air fryer basket tray with the olive oil and put the beef strips inside.
5. Cook the beef strips for 9 minutes at 365 F.
6. Stir the beef strips carefully after 4 minutes of cooking.

7. Meanwhile, wash the zucchini carefully and make spirals using a spiralizer.
8. When meat is cooked – add the zucchini spirals over the meat.
9. Sprinkle with the water, and Italian spices.
10. Cook the dish for 4 minutes more at 360 F.
11. Stir with a wooden spatula before serving.

Nutrition:
calories 226,
fat 5.3,
fiber 8,
carbs 35.25,
protein 12

Cayenne Chicken Breast
Preparation time: 20 minutes
Cooking time: 12 minutes
Servings: 4
Ingredients:

- 1-pound chicken breast, boneless, skinless
- 3 tablespoon Stevia extract
- 1 teaspoon ground white pepper
- ½ teaspoon paprika
- 1 teaspoon cayenne pepper
- 1 teaspoon lemongrass
- 1 teaspoon lemon zest
- 1 tablespoon apple cider vinegar
- 1 tablespoon butter

Directions:

1. Coat the chicken breast with the apple cider vinegar.
2. Rub the chicken breast with the ground white pepper, paprika, cayenne pepper, lemongrass, and lemon zest.
3. Leave the chicken breast for 5 minutes to marinade.
4. Rub the chicken breast with the stevia extract and leave for 5 minutes more.
5. Preheat the air fryer to 380 F.
6. Rub the Prepared chicken breast with the butter and place it in the air fryer basket tray.
7. Cook for 12 minutes turning over after 6 minutes.
8. Serve hot.

Nutrition:
calories 160, fat 5.9, fiber 0.4, carbs 1, protein 24.2

Garlic Lamb Shank
Preparation time: 15 minutes
Cooking time: 24 minutes
Servings: 5
Ingredients:

- 17 oz. lamb shanks
- 2 tablespoon garlic, peeled
- 1 teaspoon kosher salt
- 1 tablespoon dried parsley
- 4 oz chive stems, chopped
- ½ cup chicken stock
- 1 teaspoon butter
- 1 teaspoon dried rosemary
- 1 teaspoon nutmeg
- ½ teaspoon ground black pepper

Directions:

1. Chop the garlic roughly.
2. Make cuts in the lamb shank and fill with the chopped garlic.

3. Coat the lamb shank with the kosher salt, dried parsley, dried rosemary, nutmeg, and ground black pepper.
4. Stir the spices on the lamb shank gently.
5. Put the butter and chicken stock in the air fryer basket tray.
6. Preheat the air fryer to 380 F.
7. Put the chives in the air fryer basket tray.
8. Add the lamb shank and cook the meat for 24 minutes.
9. When the lamb shank is cooked, transfer it to a serving plate and sprinkle with the remaining liquid from the cooked meat.

Nutrition:
calories 205, fat 8.2,
fiber 0.8, carbs 3.8, protein 27.2

Dinner

Charred Onions and Steak Cube BBQ
Basic Recipe
Preparation Time: 5 minutes
Cooking Time: 40 minutes
Servings: 3
Ingredients:

- 1 cup red onions cut into wedges
- 1 tablespoon dry mustard
- 1 tablespoon olive oil
- 1-pound boneless beef sirloin, cut into cubes
- Salt and pepper to taste

Directions:
1. Preheat the air fryer to 390°F.
2. Place the grill pan accessory in the air fryer.
3. Toss all ingredients in a bowl and mix until everything is coated with the seasonings.
4. Place on the grill pan and cook for 40 minutes
5. Halfway through the cooking time, give a stir to cook evenly.

Nutrition:
Calories 260 Cal
Fat 10.7 g
Carbs 0 g
Protein 35.5 g

Easy Air Fried Roasted Asparagus
Basic Recipe
Preparation Time: 5 minutes
Cooking Time: 10 minutes
Servings: 4
Ingredients:

- 1 bunch fresh asparagus
- 1 ½ tsp. herbs de provence
- Fresh lemon wedge (optional)
- 1 tablespoon olive oil or cooking spray
- Salt and pepper to taste

Directions:
1. Wash asparagus and trim off hard ends. Drizzle with asparagus with olive oil and add seasonings
2. Place asparagus in air fryer and cook on 360F for 6 to 10 minutes
3. Drizzle with squeezed lemon over roasted asparagus.

Nutrition:
Calories 46
Protein 2g
Fat 3g

Carbs 1g

Air Fryer Roasted Broccoli

Basic Recipe
Preparation Time: 5 minutes
Cooking Time: 10 minutes
Servings: 4
Ingredients:

- 1 tsp. herbes de provence seasoning (optional)
- 4 cups fresh broccoli
- 1 tablespoon olive oil
- Salt and pepper to taste

Directions:

1. Drizzle with or spray broccoli with olive and sprinkle seasoning throughout
2. Spray air fryer basket with cooking oil, place broccoli and cook for 5-8 minutes on 360F
3. Open air fryer and examine broccoli after 5 minutes because different fryer brands cook at different rates.

Nutrition:
Calories 61 Fat 4g Protein 3g Carbs 4g

Air Fryer Veggie Quesadillas

Basic Recipe
Preparation Time: 20 minutes
Cooking Time: 20 minutes
Servings: 4
Ingredients:

- 4 sprouted whole-grain flour tortillas (6-in.)
- 1 cup sliced red bell pepper
- 4 ounces reduced-fat Cheddar cheese, shredded
- 1 cup sliced zucchini
- 1 cup canned black beans, Dry out and rinsed (no salt)
- Cooking spray
- 2 ounces plain 2% reduced-fat Greek yogurt
- 1 teaspoon lime zest
- 1 Tbsp. fresh juice (from 1 lime)
- ¼ tsp. ground cumin
- 2 tablespoons chopped fresh cilantro
- 1/2 cup Dry out refrigerated pico de gallo

Directions:

1. Place tortillas on work surface, sprinkle 2 tablespoons shredded cheese over half of each tortilla and top with cheese on each tortilla with 1/4 cup each red pepper slices, zucchini slices, and black beans. Sprinkle evenly with remaining 1/2 cup cheese.
2. Fold tortillas over to form half-moon shaped quesadillas, lightly coat with cooking spray, and secure with toothpicks.
3. Lightly spray air fryer basket with cooking spray. Place 2 quesadillas in the basket, and cook at 400°F for 10 minutes until tortillas are golden brown and slightly crispy, cheese is melted, and vegetables are slightly softened. Turn quesadillas over halfway through cooking.
4. Repeat with remaining quesadillas.Meanwhile, stir yogurt, lime juice, lime zest and cumin in a small bowl. Cut each quesadilla into wedges and sprinkle with cilantro.
5. Serve with 1 tablespoon cumin cream and 2 tablespoons pico de gallo each.

Nutrition:
Calories 291
Fat 8g
Protein 17g
Carbs 36g

Air Fryer Buffalo Mushroom Poppers
Basic Recipe
Preparation Time: 30 minutes
Cooking Time: 50 minutes
Servings: 8
Ingredients:

- 1-pound fresh whole button mushrooms
- 1/2 teaspoon kosher salt
- 3 tablespoons 1/3-less-fat cream cheese,
- 1/4 cup all-purpose flour
- Softened 1 jalapeño chili, seeded and minced

Cooking spray

- 1/4 teaspoon black pepper
- 1 cup panko breadcrumbs
- 2 large eggs, lightly beaten
- 1/4 cup buffalo-style hot sauce
- 2 tablespoons chopped fresh chives
- 1/2 cup low-fat buttermilk
- 1/2 cup plain fat-free yogurt
- 2 ounces blue cheese, crumbled (about 1/2 cup)
- 3 tablespoons apple cider vinegar

Directions:

1. Remove stems from mushroom caps, chop stems and set caps aside. Stir together chopped mushroom stems, cream cheese, jalapeño, salt, and pepper. Stuff about 1 teaspoon of the mixture into each mushroom cap, rounding the filling to form a smooth ball.
2. Place panko in a bowl, place flour in a second bowl, and eggs in a third Coat mushrooms in flour, dip in egg mixture, and dredge in panko, pressing to adhere. Spray mushrooms well with cooking spray.
3. Place half of the mushrooms in air fryer basket, and cook for 20 minutes at 350°F. Transfer cooked mushrooms to a large bowl. Drizzle with buffalo sauce over mushrooms; toss to coat then sprinkle with chives.
4. Stir buttermilk, yogurt, blue cheese, and cider vinegar in a small bowl. Serve mushroom poppers with blue cheese sauce.

Nutrition:
Calories 133
Fat 4g
Protein 7g
Carbs 16g

Crispy Cheesy Vegan Quesarito
Basic Recipe
Preparation Time: 5 minutes
Cooking Time: 10 minutes
Servings: 4
Ingredients:

- 2 large gluten free tortillas
- 4 tablespoons Vegan Queso (divided)
- 2-3 tablespoons grated cheese
- 3 tablespoons Meaty Crumbles
- 3-4 tablespoons cauliflower rice

- 1-2 tablespoons Spicy Almond Sauce
- 1 tablespoon cashew cream or dairy free sour cream

Added ingredients

- Fresh baby spinach, Fresh bell peppers
- Roasted red peppers

Directions:

1. Lay first tortilla flat on prep surface.
2. Cut about an inch from around the entire edge of the second tortilla using a knife, making one smaller tortilla and then set aside.
3. On the first tortilla, spread the vegan queso around the middle of the tortilla, in a circle the size of the smaller tortilla.
4. Add 3 tablespoons grated cheese to the top of the queso, in an even layer across the small circle (1 tablespoon grated cheese)
5. Top the queso / cheese circle with the smaller second tortilla, and press down slightly.
6. Spoon a line of the meaty crumbles onto the middle of the second smaller tortilla, spoon the cauliflower rice on top of the meaty crumbles, followed by the tangy cream sauce and cashew cream / sour cream.
7. Carefully fold and roll burrito tightly. Secure the edge with the reserved 1 tablespoon grated cheese. Place the burrito cheese sealed side down in air fryer basket.
8. Fry for 6-7 minutes at 370°F, or until lightly golden and crisp.

Nutrition:

Calories 514
Fat 18g
Carbs 13g
Protein 22g

Meat

Greek Vegetable Skillet
Preparation Time: 10 minutes
Cooking Time: 9 to 19 minutes
Servings: 4
Ingredients:

- ½ pound 96 percent lean ground beef
- 1 onion, chopped
- 2 garlic cloves, minced
- 2 cups fresh baby spinach (see Tip)
- 2 tablespoons freshly squeezed lemon juice
- ⅓ cup low-sodium beef broth
- 2 tablespoons crumbled low-sodium feta cheese

Directions:

1. In a 6-by-2-inch metal pan, crumble the beef. Cook in the air fryer for 3 to 7 minutes, stirring once during cooking, until browned. Drain off any fat or liquid.
2. Add the onion, and garlic to the pan. Air-fry for 4 to 8 minutes more, or until the onion is tender.
3. Add the spinach, lemon juice, and beef broth. Air-fry for 2 to 4 minutes more, or until the spinach is wilted.
4. Sprinkle with the feta cheese and serve immediately

Nutrition:

Calories: 97
Fat: 1g
 Saturated Fat: 1g
Protein: 15g
Carbohydrates: 5g
Sodium: 123mg
Fiber: 1g
Sugar: 2g

Light Herbed Meatballs

Preparation Time: 10 minutes
Cooking Time: 12 to 17 minutes
Servings: 24
Ingredients:

- 1 medium onion, minced
- 2 garlic cloves, minced
- 1 teaspoon olive oil
- 1 slice low-sodium whole-wheat bread, crumbled
- 3 tablespoons 1 percent milk
- 1 teaspoon dried marjoram
- 1 teaspoon dried basil
- 1-pound 96 percent lean ground beef

Directions:

1. In a 6-by-2-inch pan, combine the onion, garlic, and olive oil. Air-fry for 2 to 4 minutes, or until the vegetables are crisp-tender.
2. Transfer the vegetables to a medium bowl, and add the bread crumbs, milk, marjoram, and basil. Mix well.
3. Add the ground beef. With your hands, work the mixture gently but thoroughly until combined. Form the meat mixture into about 24 (1-inch) meatballs.
4. Bake the meatballs, in batches, in the air fryer basket for 12 to 17 minutes, or until they reach 160°F

on a meat thermometer. Serve immediately.

Nutrition:
Calories: 190
Fat: 6g
Saturated Fat: 2g
Protein: 25g
Carbohydrates: 8g
Sodium: 120mg
Fiber: 1g;
Sugar: 2g
1% DV vitamin A
3% DV vitamin C

Cauliflower Rice And Beef-Stuffed Bell Peppers

Preparation Time: 10 minutes
Cooking Time: 11 to 16 minutes
Servings: 4
Ingredients:

- 4 medium bell peppers, any colors, rinsed, tops removed
- 1 medium onion, chopped
- ½ cup grated carrot
- 2 teaspoons olive oil
- 1 cup cooked cauliflower rice
- 1 cup chopped cooked low-sodium roast beef
- 1 teaspoon dried marjoram

Directions:

1. Remove the stems from the bell pepper tops and chop the tops.
2. In a 6-by-2-inch pan, combine the chopped bell pepper tops, onion, carrot, and olive oil. Cook for 2 to 4 minutes, or until the vegetables are crisp-tender.
3. Transfer the vegetables to a medium bowl. Add the cauliflower rice, roast beef, and marjoram. Stir to mix.

4. Stuff the vegetable mixture into the bell peppers. Place the bell peppers in the air fryer basket. Bake for 11 to 16 minutes, or until the peppers are tender and the filling is hot. Serve immediately.

Nutrition:
Calories: 206
Fat: 6g
Saturated Fat: 1g
 Protein: 18g
Carbohydrates: 20g
Sodium: 105mg
Fiber: 3g
Sugar: 5g

Fish

Baked Basa
Preparation Time: 10 minutes
Cooking Time: 30 minutes
Servings: 2
Ingredients:

- 2 basa fish fillets
- 4 lemon slices
- 1/8 teaspoon lemon juice
- 1/2 tablespoon dried basil
- 1/2 teaspoon paprika
- 4 teaspoon butter, melted
- 1/8 teaspoon salt

Directions:

1. In a small bowl, mix together butter, paprika, basil, lemon juice, and salt.
2. Brush fish fillets with melted butter mixture.
3. Place the cooking tray in the air fryer basket. Line air fryer basket with parchment paper.
4. Select Air Fry mode.
5. Set time to 30 minutes and temperature 350 F then press START.
6. The air fryer display will prompt you to ADD FOOD once the temperature is reached then place fish fillets in the air fryer basket and place lemon slices on fish fillets.
7. Turn fish fillets halfway through.
8. Serve and enjoy.

Nutrition:
Calories 293 Fat 19.6 g
Carbohydrates 5.8 g Sugar 3.2 g
Protein 24 g
Cholesterol 20 mg

Parmesan Cod
Preparation Time: 10 minutes
Cooking Time: 15 minutes
Servings: 4
Ingredients:

- 4 cod fillets
- 1 tablespoon olive oil
- 1 tablespoon parsley, chopped
- 2 teaspoon paprika
- 3/4 cup parmesan cheese, grated
- 1/4 teaspoon sea salt

Directions:

1. In a shallow dish, mix together parmesan cheese, paprika, parsley, and salt.

2. Brush fish fillets with oil and coat with cheese mixture.
3. Place the cooking tray in the air fryer basket. Line air fryer basket with parchment paper.
4. Select Bake mode.
5. Set time to 15 minutes and temperature 400 F then press START.
6. The air fryer display will prompt you to ADD FOOD once the temperature is reached then place the fish fillet in the air fryer basket.
7. Serve and enjoy.

Nutrition:
Calories 265
Fat 14.1 g
Carbohydrates 2.2 g
Sugar 0.1 g
Protein 34.3 g
Cholesterol 86 mg

Lemon Pepper Tilapia

Preparation Time: 10 minutes
Cooking Time: 15 minutes
Servings: 4
Ingredients:

- 4 tilapia fillets, thawed
- 4 tablespoon lemon pepper seasoning

Directions:

1. Spray fish fillets with cooking spray.
2. Sprinkle lemon pepper seasoning over fish fillets.
3. Place the cooking tray in the air fryer basket. Line air fryer basket with parchment paper.
4. Select Bake mode.

5. Set time to 15 minutes and temperature 350 F then press START.
6. The air fryer display will prompt you to ADD FOOD once the temperature is reached then place the fish fillet in the air fryer basket.
7. Serve and enjoy.

Nutrition:
Calories 109
Fat 1.2 g
Carbohydrates 4.2 g
Sugar 0 g
Protein 21.7 g
Cholesterol 55 mg

<u>Vegetable</u>

Squash Noodles

Preparation Time: 10 minutes
Cooking Time: 25 minutes
Servings: 2
Ingredients:

- 1 medium butternut squash, peel and spiralized
- 3 tablespoon cream
- 1/4 cup parmesan cheese
- 1 teaspoon thyme, chopped
- 1 tablespoon sage, chopped
- 1 teaspoon garlic powder
- 2 tablespoon cream cheese

Directions:

1. In a bowl, mix together cream cheese, parmesan, thyme, sage, cream, and garlic powder.
2. Add noodles to a baking dish.
3. Select Bake mode.

4. Set time to 20 minutes and temperature 400 F then press START.
5. The air fryer display will prompt you to ADD FOOD once the temperature is reached then place the baking dish in the air fryer basket.
6. Spread the cream cheese mixture over noodles and bake for 5 minutes more.
7. Serve and enjoy.

Nutrition:
Calories 180 Fat 11 g
Carbohydrates 12 g Sugar 2.3 g
Protein 11.3 g
Cholesterol 35 mg

Cheesy Zucchini Noodles

Preparation Time: 10 minutes
Cooking Time: 45 minutes
Servings: 3
Ingredients:

- 1 egg
- 2 medium zucchini, trimmed and spiralized
- 1/2 cup parmesan cheese, grated
- 1/2 cup feta cheese, crumbled
- 2 tablespoon olive oil
- 1 cup mozzarella cheese, grated
- 1 tablespoon thyme
- 1 garlic clove, chopped
- 1 onion, chopped
- 1/2 teaspoon pepper
- 1/2 teaspoon salt

Directions:

1. Add spiralized zucchini and salt in a colander and set aside for 10 minutes.
2. Gently wash zucchini noodles and pat dry with a paper towel.
3. Heat oil in a pan over medium heat. Add garlic and onion and sauté for 3-4 minutes.
4. Add zucchini noodles and cook for 4 minutes or until softened.
5. Add zucchini mixture into a baking dish add the eggs, thyme, cheeses. Mix well and season with pepper and salt.
6. Select Bake mode.
7. Set time to 45 minutes and temperature 375 F then press START.
8. The air fryer display will prompt you to ADD FOOD once the temperature is reached then place the baking dish in the air fryer basket.
9. Serve and enjoy.

Nutrition:
Calories 359 Fat 26.5 g
Carbohydrates 11.8 g
Sugar 5 g
Protein 22.8 g
Cholesterol 110 mg

Roasted Carrots

Preparation Time: 10 minutes
Cooking Time: 35 minutes
Servings: 6
Ingredients:

- 16 small carrots
- 1 tablespoon fresh parsley, chopped
- 1 tablespoon dried basil
- 6 garlic cloves, minced
- 4 tablespoon olive oil
- 1 1/2 teaspoon salt

Directions:

1. In a bowl, combine together oil, carrots, basil, garlic, and salt.
2. Spread the carrots into a baking dish.
3. Select Bake mode.
4. Set time to 35 minutes and temperature 375 F then press START.
5. The air fryer display will prompt you to ADD FOOD once the temperature is reached then place the baking dish in the air fryer basket.
6. Garnish with parsley and serve.

Nutrition:
Calories 94
Fat 9.4 g
Carbohydrates 3.2 g
Sugar 1.3 g
Protein 0.4 g
Cholesterol 0 mg

Roasted Cauliflower and Broccoli

Preparation Time: 10 minutes
Cooking Time: 20 minutes
Servings: 6
Ingredients:

- 4 cups broccoli florets
- 4 cups cauliflower florets
- 2/3 cup parmesan cheese, shredded
- 1/3 cup olive oil
- 3 garlic cloves, minced
- Pepper
- Salt

Directions:

1. Add half parmesan cheese, broccoli, cauliflower, garlic, oil, pepper, and salt into the large bowl and toss well.
2. Spread broccoli and cauliflower mixture in a baking dish.
3. Select Bake mode.
4. Set time to 20 minutes and temperature 400 F then press START.
5. The air fryer display will prompt you to ADD FOOD once the temperature is reached then place the baking dish in the air fryer basket.
6. Add remaining cheese and toss well.
7. Serve and enjoy.

Nutrition:
Calories 220
Fat 17.1 g
Carbohydrates 9 g
Sugar 2.7 g
Protein 11.5 g
Cholesterol 19 mg

Snacks

Parmesan Turnip Slices

Preparation time: 12 minutes
Cooking time: 10 minutes
Servings: 8
Ingredients:

- 1 teaspoon garlic powder
- 1-pound turnip
- 1 teaspoon salt
- 3 oz. Parmesan, shredded
- 1 tablespoon olive oil

Directions:

1. Peel the turnip and slice it.
2. Sprinkle the sliced turnip with salt and garlic powder.
3. Drizzle the turnip slices with olive oil.
4. Preheat the air fryer to 360 F.
5. Put the turnip slices in the air fryer basket and cook them for 10 minutes.
6. Serve.

Nutrition:
calories 66,
fat 4.1,
fiber 1.1,
carbs 4.3,
protein 4

Salty Cucumber Chips

Preparation time: 10 minutes
Cooking time: 11 minutes
Servings: 12
Ingredients:

- 1-pound cucumber
- 1 teaspoon salt
- 1 tablespoon smoked paprika
- ½ teaspoon garlic powder

Directions:

1. Wash the cucumbers carefully and slice them into chips.
2. Sprinkle the chips with salt, smoked paprika, and garlic powder.
3. Preheat the air fryer to 370 F.
4. Place the cucumber slices in the air fryer rack.
5. Cook the cucumber chips for 11 minutes.
6. Transfer the cucumber chips to a paper towel and allow to cool.
7. Serve the cucumber chips immediately or keep them in a paper bag.

Nutrition:
calories 8,
fat 0.1,
fiber 0.4,
carbs 1.8,
protein 0.4

Spinach Balls with Chicken

Preparation time: 15 minutes
Cooking time: 11 minutes
Servings: 7
Ingredients:

- 4 large eggs
- 1 cup spinach
- ½ teaspoon salt
- 1 tablespoon minced garlic
- 8 oz. ground chicken
- 2 tablespoon almond flour
- 1 teaspoon olive oil

- 1 teaspoon smoked paprika
- 1 teaspoon coconut flour

Directions:

1. Crack the eggs and transfer them to a blender.

2. Add the spinach, salt, minced garlic, almond flour, smoked paprika, and coconut flour.

3. Blend until well combined.

4. Transfer the mixture into a bowl.

5. Add the ground chicken and stir.

6. Make your hands wet and make medium balls from the spinach mixture.

7. Preheat the air fryer to 370 F.

8. Grease the air fryer basket with olive oil.

9. Put the spinach balls in the air fryer and cook for 11 minutes.

10. Serve the snack immediately or keep it in a plastic container in the fridge.

Nutrition:
calories 159, fat 10, fiber 1.2, carbs 2.9, protein 15

Eggplant Chips

Preparation time: 15 minutes
Cooking time: 13 minutes
Servings: 10
Ingredients:

- 1 teaspoon onion powder
- 1 teaspoon salt
- 3 eggplants
- 1 teaspoon paprika
- ½ teaspoon ground black pepper
- 1 tablespoon olive oil

Directions:

1. Wash the eggplants and slice them into chips.

2. Sprinkle the eggplant slices with salt and let it absorb the eggplant juice and bitterness.

3. Dry the eggplant slices and sprinkle them with onion powder, paprika, and ground black pepper.

4. Stir the eggplant slices using your fingertips.

5. Then preheat the air fryer to 400 F.

6. Place the eggplant slices in the air fryer rack and cook them for 13 minutes. The temperature of cooking depends on the thickness of the eggplant slices.

Nutrition:
calories 46, fat 1.4, fiber 5.3, carbs 8.2, protein 1.1

Dessert

Sweet Baked Avocado

Preparation Time: 5 minutes
Cooking time: 20 minutes
Servings: 2
Ingredients:

- 1 avocado, pitted, halved
- 2 teaspoons Erythritol
- 1 teaspoon vanilla extract
- 2 teaspoons butter

Directions:

1. Sprinkle the avocado halves with Erythritol, vanilla extract, and butter.
2. Put the avocado halves in the air fryer and cook at 350F for 20 minutes.

Nutrition:

calories 245,

fat 23.4,

fiber 6.7,

carbs 8.9,

protein 2

Avocado Cream

Preparation Time: 10 minutes
Cooking time: 30 minutes
Servings: 5
Ingredients:

- 1 avocado, peeled, pitted, chopped
- 1 egg, beaten
- 2 tablespoon Erythritol
- 1 cup coconut cream
- 1 tablespoon butter, softened
- ½ teaspoon ground nutmeg

Directions:

1. Blend the avocado with egg, Erythritol, coconut cream, butter, and ground nutmeg.
2. When the liquid is smooth, transfer it in the ramekins.
3. Put the ramekins in the air fryer basket and cook at 345F for 30 minutes.

Nutrition:

calories 227,

fat 22.5,

fiber 3.8,

carbs 6.3,

protein 3

Sesame Seeds Cookies

Preparation time: 15 minutes
Cooking time: 10 minutes
Servings: 8
Ingredients:

- 1 cup almond flour
- 2 tablespoons coconut shred
- 2 eggs, beaten
- 1 teaspoon baking powder
- ¼ cup Splenda
- 3 tablespoons sesame seeds
- 1 tablespoon coconut oil, softened

Directions:

1. Put all ingredients in the mixing bowl and knead the dough.
2. Make the balls from the dough and press them gently in the shape of the cookies.
3. Put the cookies in the air fryer basket in one layer and cook them for 10 minutes at 360F.

Nutrition:

calories 177,

fat 12.4,

fiber 2.2,

carbs 10.7,

protein 5

Walnut Bars

Preparation Time: 15 minutes
Cooking time: 16 minutes
Servings: 4
Ingredients:

- 1 egg, beaten
- 2 tablespoons Erythritol
- 7 tablespoons coconut oil, softened
- 1 teaspoon vanilla extract
- ¼ cup coconut flour

- 1 oz walnuts, chopped
- ½ teaspoon baking powder

Directions:

1. Mix egg with Erythritol, coconut oil, vanilla extract, coconut flour, and baking powder.
2. Stir the mixture gently, add walnuts, and mix the mixture until homogenous.
3. Pour the mixture in the air fryer basket and flatten gently.
4. Cook the walnut bars at 375F for 16 minutes.
5. Cool the dessert well and cut into bars.

Nutrition:
calories 298,
fat 29.8,
fiber 3.5,
carbs 6.2,
protein 4.1

Keto Blondies

Preparation time: 10 minutes
Cooking time: 15 minutes
Servings: 2
Ingredients:

- 1 egg, beaten
- 1 tablespoon almond butter
- ½ teaspoon baking powder
- 1 teaspoon lime juice
- ½ teaspoon vanilla extract
- 1 teaspoon Splenda
- 2 tablespoons almond flour

Directions:

1. Put all ingredients in the mixer bowl and mix until smooth.
2. Pour the mixture in the air fryer basket, flatten gently, and cook at 375F for 15 minutes.
3. Then cut the cooked dessert into servings.

Nutrition:
calories 138,
fat 10.1,
fiber 1.6,
carbs 6.4,
protein 6

Chocolate Cream

Preparation Time: 10 minutes
Cooking time: 15 minutes
Servings: 3
Ingredients:

- 1 oz dark chocolate, chopped
- 1 cup coconut cream
- 1 teaspoon vanilla extract
- 1 tablespoon Erythritol

Directions:

1. Pour coconut cream in the air fryer.
2. Add chocolate, vanilla extract, and Erythritol.
3. Cook the chocolate cream for 15 minutes at 360F. Stir the liquid from time to time during cooking.

Nutrition:
calories 236,
fat 21.9,
fiber 2,
carbs 10.3,
protein 2.6

CHAPTER 13:

November

Lunch

Turmeric Pork Bites

Preparation time: 15 minutes
Cooking time: 14 minutes
Servings: 6
Ingredients:

- 1-pound pork brisket
- 6 oz. bacon, sliced
- 1 teaspoon salt
- 1 teaspoon turmeric
- ½ teaspoon red pepper
- 1 teaspoon olive oil
- 1 tablespoon apple cider vinegar

Directions:

1. Cut the pork brisket into medium bites.
2. Put the pork bites in the big mixing bowl.
3. Sprinkle the meat with the turmeric, salt, red pepper, and apple cider vinegar.
4. Mix the pork bites carefully and leave them for 10 minutes to marinade.
5. Wrap the pork bites in the sliced bacon.
6. Secure the pork bites with the toothpicks.
7. Preheat the air fryer to 370 F.
8. Put the Prepared bacon pork bites on the air fryer tray.
9. Cook the pork bites for 8 minutes.
10. Turn the pork over.
11. Cook the dish for 6 minutes more.

Nutrition:
calories 239,
fat 13.7,
fiber 0.2,
carbs 2.8,
protein 26.8

Cheddar Salmon Casserole

Preparation time: 20 minutes
Cooking time: 12 minutes
Servings: 8
Ingredients:

- 7 oz Cheddar cheese, shredded
- ½ cup cream
- 1-pound salmon fillet
- 1 tablespoon dried dill
- 1 teaspoon dried parsley
- 1 teaspoon salt
- 1 teaspoon ground coriander
- ½ teaspoon ground black pepper
- 2 green pepper, chopped

- 4 oz chive stems, diced
- 7 oz bok choy, chopped
- 1 tablespoon olive oil

Directions:

1. Coat the salmon fillet with the dried dill, dried parsley, ground coriander, and ground black pepper.
2. Massage the salmon fillet gently and leave it for 5 minutes to marinate.
3. Meanwhile, grease the air fryer casserole tray with the olive oil.
4. Cut the salmon fillet into the cubes.
5. Separate the salmon cubes into 2 portions.
6. Place the first portion of salmon cubes in the casserole tray.
7. Sprinkle the fish with the chopped bok choy, diced chives, and chopped green pepper.
8. Then place the second portion of salmon cubes over the vegetables.
9. Sprinkle the casserole with the shredded cheese and heavy cream.
10. Preheat the air fryer to 380 F.
11. Cook the salmon casserole for 12 minutes.
12. When the dish is cooked – it will have a crunchy light brown crust.

Nutrition:
calories 216, fat 14.4,
fiber 1.1, carbs 4.3,
protein 18.2

Indian Lamb Meatballs

Preparation time: 10 minutes
Cooking time: 14 minutes
Servings: 8
Ingredients:

- 1 garlic clove
- 1 tablespoon butter
- 4 oz chive stems
- ¼ tablespoon turmeric
- 1/3 teaspoon cayenne pepper
- 1 teaspoon ground coriander
- ¼ teaspoon bay leaf
- 1 teaspoon salt
- 1-pound ground lamb
- 1 egg
- 1 teaspoon ground black pepper

Directions:

1. Peel the garlic clove and mince it
2. Combine the minced garlic with the ground lamb.
3. Coat the meat mixture with the turmeric, cayenne pepper, ground coriander, bay leaf, salt, and ground black pepper.
4. Crack the egg in the meat.
5. Finely chop the chives and add them in the lamb.
6. Mix well to combine.
7. Preheat the air fryer to 400 F.
8. Put the butter in the air fryer basket tray and melt it.
9. Make the meatballs from the lamb mixture and place them in the air fryer basket tray.

10. Cook for 14 minutes, stirring occasionally.

Nutrition:
calories 134,
fat 6.2,
fiber 0.4,
carbs 1.8,
protein 16.9

Korean Beef Bowl

Preparation time: 15 minutes
Cooking time: 18 minutes
Servings: 4
Ingredients:

- 1 tablespoon minced garlic
- 1 teaspoon ground ginger
- 4 oz chive stems, chopped
- 2 tablespoon apple cider vinegar
- 1 teaspoon stevia extract
- 1 tablespoon flax seeds
- 1 teaspoon olive oil
- 1 teaspoon olive oil
- 1-pound ground beef
- 4 tablespoon chicken stock

Directions:

1. Coat the ground beef with the apple cider vinegar and stir the meat with a spoon.
2. Add the ground ginger, minced garlic, and olive oil.
3. Mix well.
4. Preheat the air fryer to 370 F.
5. Put the ground beef in the air fryer basket tray and cook for 8 minutes.
6. Stir the ground beef carefully and sprinkle with the chopped chives, flax seeds, olive oil, and chicken stock.

7. Mix well and cook for 10 minutes more.
8. Stir and serve hot.

Nutrition:
calories 258,
fat 10.1,
fiber 1.2,
carbs 4.2,
protein 35.3

Keto Lamb Kleftiko

Preparation time: 25 minutes
Cooking time: 30 minutes
Servings: 6
Ingredients:

- 2 oz. garlic clove, peeled
- 1 tablespoon dried oregano
- ½ lemon
- ¼ tablespoon ground cinnamon
- 3 tablespoon butter, frozen
- 18 oz. leg of lamb
- 1 cup heavy cream
- 1 teaspoon bay leaf
- 1 teaspoon dried mint
- 1 tablespoon olive oil

Directions:

1. Crush the garlic cloves and combine them with the dried oregano, and ground cinnamon.
2. Chop the lemon.
3. Coat the leg of lamb with the crushed garlic mixture.
4. Rub it with the chopped lemon.
5. Combine the heavy cream, bay leaf, and dried mint together.
6. Whisk the mixture well.

7. Add the olive oil and whisk it one more time more.
8. Pour the cream mixture on the leg of lamb and stir it carefully.
9. Leave the leg of lamb for 10 minutes to marinade.
10. Preheat the air fryer to 380 F.
11. Chop the butter and coat over the lamb.
12. Place the leg of lamb in the air fryer basket tray and coat it with the remaining cream mixture.
13. Then add the chopped butter over the meat.
14. Cook for 30 minutes.
15. Remove the meat from the air fryer and sprinkle it gently with the remaining cream mixture. Serve hot.

Nutrition:
calories 318,
fat 21.9,
fiber 0.9,
carbs 4.9,
protein 25.1

Pork Chops with Keto Gravy
Preparation time: 15 minutes
Cooking time: 17 minutes
Servings: 4
Ingredients:
- 1-pound pork chops
- 1 teaspoon kosher salt
- ½ teaspoon ground cinnamon
- 1 teaspoon ground white pepper
- 1 cup heavy cream
- 6 oz. white mushrooms
- 1 tablespoon butter
- ½ teaspoon ground ginger
- 1 teaspoon ground turmeric
- 4 oz chive stems
- 1 garlic clove, chopped

Directions:
1. Coat the pork chops with the kosher salt, ground cinnamon, ground white pepper, and ground turmeric.
2. Preheat the air fryer to 375 F.
3. Pour the heavy cream in the air fryer basket tray.
4. Slice the white mushrooms and add them to the heavy cream.
5. Add butter, ground ginger, chopped chives, and chopped garlic.
6. Cook for 5 minutes.
7. Stir and add the pork chops.
8. Cook the pork chops at 400 F for 12 minutes.
9. Stir the pork chops gently and transfer to a serving plate.

Nutrition:
calories 518, fat 42.4,
fiber 1.5, carbs 6.2,
protein 28

Cinnamon Pork Tenderloin
Preparation time: 20 minutes
Cooking time: 15 minutes
Servings: 3
Ingredients:
- ½ teaspoon saffron
- 1 teaspoon sage

- ½ teaspoon ground cinnamon
- 1 teaspoon garlic powder
- 1 teaspoon onion powder
- 1-pound pork tenderloin
- 3 tablespoon butter
- 1 garlic clove, crushed
- 1 tablespoon apple cider vinegar

Directions:

1. Combine the saffron, sage, ground cinnamon, garlic powder, and onion powder together in a shallow bowl.
2. Mix the spices well to combine.
3. Coat the pork tenderloin in the spice mixture.
4. Rub the pork tenderloin with the crushed garlic and coat the meat with the apple cider vinegar.
5. Leave the pork tenderloin for 10 minutes to marinade.
6. Meanwhile, preheat the air fryer to 320 F.
7. Put the pork tenderloin in the air fryer tray and place the butter over the meat.
8. Cook for 15 minutes.
9. Allow the meat to rest briefly.
10. Slice the pork tenderloin and serve.

Nutrition:
calories 328,
fat 16.9,
fiber 0.5,
carbs 2.2,
protein 40

Rosemary Duck Legs

Preparation time: 25 minutes
Cooking time: 25 minutes
Servings: 6
Ingredients:

- 1 lemon
- 2-pound duck legs
- 1 teaspoon ground coriander
- 1 teaspoon ground nutmeg
- 1 teaspoon kosher salt
- ½ teaspoon dried rosemary
- 1 tablespoon olive oil
- 1 teaspoon stevia extract
- ¼ teaspoon sage

Directions:

1. Squeeze the juice from the lemon and grate the zest.
2. Combine the lemon juice and lemon zest together in a large mixing bowl.
3. Add the ground coriander, ground nutmeg, kosher salt, dried rosemary, and sage.
4. Add the olive oil and stevia extract.
5. Whisk carefully and add the duck legs.
6. Stir the duck legs and leave them for 15 minutes to marinade.
7. Preheat the air fryer to 380 F.
8. Put the marinated duck legs in the air fryer and cook for 25 minutes, turning after 15 minutes.
9. Allow the duck to rest before serving.

Nutrition:
calories 296, fat 11.5, fiber 0.5,
carbs 1.6, protein 44.2

Chili Pepper Lamb Chops

Preparation time: 20 minutes
Cooking time: 10 minutes
Servings: 6
Ingredients:

- 21 oz. lamb chops
- 1 teaspoon chili pepper
- ½ teaspoon chili flakes
- 1 teaspoon onion powder
- 1 teaspoon garlic powder
- 1 teaspoon cayenne pepper
- 1 tablespoon olive oil
- 1 tablespoon butter
- ½ teaspoon lime zest

Directions:

1. Melt the butter and combine it with the olive oil.
2. Whisk then add chili pepper, chili flakes, onion powder, garlic powder, cayenne pepper, and lime zest.
3. Mix well.
4. Coat the lamb chops with the marinade.
5. Leave the meat for at least 5 minutes in the fridge.
6. Preheat the air fryer to 400 F.
7. Place the marinated lamb chops in the air fryer and cook them for 5 minutes.
8. Turn the chops over.
9. Cook the lamb chops for 5 minutes more.

Nutrition:
calories 227,
fat 11.6,
fiber 0.2,
carbs 1,
protein 28.1

Creamy Kebab

Preparation time: 15 minutes
Cooking time: 10 minutes
Servings: 5
Ingredients:

- 14 oz. chicken fillet
- ½ cup heavy cream
- 1 teaspoon kosher salt
- ½ teaspoon ground black pepper
- 1 teaspoon turmeric
- 1 teaspoon curry powder
- 1 teaspoon olive oil

Directions:

1. Combine the heavy cream with the kosher salt, ground black pepper, turmeric, and curry powder.
2. Whisk the mixture well.
3. Add oil and whisk again.
4. Cut the chicken fillet into pieces.
5. Add the chicken to the heavy cream mixture and stir carefully.
6. Preheat the air fryer to 360 F.
7. Put the chicken kebab in the air fryer rack and cook it for 10 minutes.

Nutrition:
calories 204,
fat 11.4,
fiber 0.3,
carbs 1,
protein 23.3

Beef Meatballs

Preparation time: 15 minutes
Cooking time: 11 minutes
Servings: 6
Ingredients:

- 1 tablespoon almond flour
- 1-pound ground beef
- 1 teaspoon dried parsley
- 1 teaspoon dried dill
- ½ teaspoon ground nutmeg
- 1 oz chive stems
- 1 teaspoon garlic powder
- 1 teaspoon salt
- ½ cup heavy cream
- ¼ cup chicken stock
- 1 teaspoon mustard
- 1 teaspoon ground black pepper
- 1 tablespoon butter

Directions:

1. Combine the ground beef and almond flour together in the bowl.
2. Add the dried dill, dried parsley, ground nutmeg, garlic powder, chopped chives, salt, ground black pepper, and mustard.
3. Mix well to combine.
4. Make the meatballs from the mixture.
5. Preheat the air fryer to 380 F.
6. Put the meatballs in the air fryer basket tray.
7. Add the butter and cook the dish for 5 minutes.
8. Turn the meatballs over.
9. Coat the meatballs with the heavy cream and chicken stock.
10. Cook for 6 minutes more.
11. Serve immediately with the cream gravy.

Nutrition:
calories 227,
fat 12.9,
fiber 0.9,
carbs 2.7,
protein 24.6

Dinner

Chicken Veggie Fritters

Preparation Time: 10 minutes

Cooking Time: 25 minutes

Serve: 4

Ingredients:

- 1 lb ground chicken
- 3/4 cup almond flour
- 1 egg, lightly beaten
- 1 garlic clove, minced
- 1 1/2 cup mozzarella cheese, shredded
- 1/2 cup shallots, chopped
- 2 cups broccoli, chopped
- Pepper
- Salt

Directions:

1. Add all ingredients into the large bowl and mix until well combined.
2. Make small patties from mixture and place onto the parchment-lined cooking tray.
3. Select BAKE mode, then set the temperature to 390 F and the time to 25 minutes, then press start.
4. When the display shows Add Food then place the cooking tray in the vortex plus air fryer oven.
5. Turn chicken patties halfway through.
6. Serve and enjoy.

Nutrition:

Calories 412

Fat 22.1 g

Carbohydrates 11.6 g

Sugar 1.6 g

Protein 43.5 g

Cholesterol 147 mg

Cheese and Veggie Cups
Basic Recipe
Preparation Time: 10 minutes
Cooking Time: 20 minutes
Servings: 4
Ingredients:
- Non-stick cooking spray
- 4 large eggs
- 1 cup diced veggies of choice
- 1 cup shredded cheese
- 4 Tbsp. half and half
- 1 Tbsp. chopped cilantro
- Salt and Pepper

Directions:
1. Grease 4 ramekins
2. Whisk eggs, vegetables, half the cheese, half and half, cilantro, and salt and pepper together. In a medium bowl and divide between the ramekins
3. Place ramekins in the air-fryer basket, set temperature to 300 F for 12 minutes
4. Top the cups with remaining cheese.
5. Set air-fryer to 400 degrees F, cook 2 minutes until cheese is melted.

Nutrition:
Calories 195kcal
Carbs 7g
Protein 13g
Fat 12g

Air Fryer Vegetables
Basic Recipe
Preparation Time: 5 minutes
Cooking Time: 10 minutes
Servings: 4
Ingredients:
- 1/2 lb. broccoli fresh
- 1/2 lb. cauliflower fresh
- 1 tbsp.olive oil
- 1/4 tsp. seasoning
- 1/3 c water

Directions:
1. Mix vegetables, olive oil and seasonings in a medium bowl.

2. Pour 1/3 c. water in the Air Fryer base to prevent from smoking.
3. Place vegetables in the air fryer basket.
4. Cook at 400 degrees for 7-10 minutes
5. Shake vegetables half way through the 7-10 minutes

Nutrition:
Calories 65kcal
Carbs 7g
Protein 3g
Fat 4g

Mushroom, Onion and Feta Frittata
Basic Recipe
Preparation Time: 15 minutes
Cooking Time: 10 minutes
Servings: 4
Ingredients:
- 3 whole eggs
- 2 cup sliced button mushrooms
- ½ red onions
- 1 tbsp. Olive oil
- 3 tbspcrumbled feta
- 1 pinch salt

Directions:
1. Peel and slice half a red onion into ¼ inch thin slices.
2. Wash button mushrooms; then slice into ¼ inch thin slices.
3. Place a pan under a medium flame, add olive oil sweat onions and mushrooms and sauté until tender.Take onions and mushrooms off the heat and place on kitchen towel to cool.
4. Preheat Air fryer to 320°F.
5. In a mixing bowl crack 3 eggs and whisk thoroughly and vigorously.

6. Coat the outside and bottom of a 6-ounce ramekin lightly with pan spray.
7. Pour eggs into the ramekin, add ¼ cup onion and mushrooms mixture, and then add cheese.
8. Place in Air fryer and cook for 10 to 12 minutes

Nutrition:
Calories 90
Fat 4.5g
Carbs 8g
Protein 13g

Sweet and Spicy Air Fryer Brussels Sprouts
Basic Recipe
Preparation Time: 5 minutes
Cooking Time: 20 minutes
Servings: 8
Ingredients:
- 1 Brussels sprout cut into two halves
- 1 ½ tablespoon vegetable oil
- ½ tsp. salt
- 2 tablespoon honey
- 1 tablespoon gochujang

Directions:
1. Mix honey, gochujang, vegetable oil and salt in a bowl and stir properly. Take out 1 tablespoon of the sauce and set it aside then add Brussels sprout to the bowl and stir until the sprout is mixed properly
2. Place the Brussels sprouts into your Air fryer, set heat at 360ºF and cook for 15 minutes; shake the basket halfway into cooking time and set the bowl aside when the timer is off.

3. When the timer goes off, increase the temperature to 390ºF and cook for another 5 minutes

After 5 minute, put sprouts in a bowl and cover with reserved sauce and stir.

Nutrition:

Calories 128

Fat 4g

Carbs 20g

Protein 3g

Roasted Air Fryer Sweet Carrots

Basic Recipe

Preparation Time: 10 minutes

Cooking Time: 20 minutes

Servings: 4

Ingredients:

- 1 lb. carrots, peeled and chopped into 1-inch pieces
- ¼ tablespoons salt
- 2 tablespoons brown sugar
- 2 tablespoons melted butter

Directions:

1. Place peeled and chopped carrots in a bowl, add melted butter, brown sugar and salt and stir properly until the carrot is properly coated.
2. Pour coated mixture into an air fryer safe bowl, place it in the air fryer, set heat at 380º F and cook for 10 minutes, stir and cook for another 10 minutes
3. Your sweet carrot is ready to be served.

Nutrition:

Calcium 42mg

Vitamin 7mg

Fiber 3g

Carbs 17g

Sodium 275mg

Meat

Beef And Broccoli

Preparation Time: 10 minutes

Cooking Time: 14 to 18 minutes

Servings: 4

Ingredients:

- 2 tablespoons glucomannan
- ½ cup low-sodium beef broth
- 1 teaspoon low-sodium soy sauce
- 12 ounces sirloin strip steak, cut into 1-inch cubes
- 2½ cups broccoli florets
- 1 onion, chopped
- 1 cup sliced cremini mushrooms
- 1 tablespoon grated fresh ginger
- Cauliflower rice, cooked (optional)

Directions:

1. In a medium bowl, stir together the glucomannan, beef broth, and soy sauce.
2. Add the beef and toss to coat. Let stand for 5 minutes at room temperature.
3. With a slotted spoon, transfer the beef from the broth mixture into a medium metal bowl. Reserve the broth.
4. Add the broccoli, onion, mushrooms, and ginger to the beef. Place the bowl into the air fryer and cook for 12 to 15 minutes, or until the beef reaches at least 145°F on a meat thermometer and the vegetables are tender.
5. Add the reserved broth and cook for 2 to 3 minutes more, or until the sauce boils.

6. Serve immediately over hot cooked cauliflower rice, if desired.

Nutrition:
Calories: 240
Fat: 6g
Saturated Fat: 2g
Protein: 19g
Carbohydrates: 11g
 Sodium: 107mg
Fiber: 2g
Sugar: 3g

Beef And Fruit Stir-Fry
Preparation Time: 15 minutes
Cooking Time: 6 to 11 minutes
Servings: 4
Ingredients:

- 12 ounces sirloin tip steak, thinly sliced
- 1 tablespoon freshly squeezed lime juice
- 1 cup canned mandarin orange segments, drained, juice reserved
- 1 teaspoon low-sodium soy sauce
- 1 tablespoon glucomannan
- 1 teaspoon olive oil
- 2 scallions, white and green parts, sliced
- cauliflower rice, cooked (optional)

Directions:
1. In a medium bowl, mix the steak with the lime juice. Set aside.
2. In a small bowl, thoroughly mix 3 tablespoons of reserved mandarin orange juice, the soy sauce, and glucomannan.
3. Drain the beef and transfer it to a medium metal bowl, reserving the juice. Stir the reserved juice into the mandarin juice mixture. Set aside.

4. Add the olive oil and scallions to the steak. Place the metal bowl in the air fryer and cook for 3 to 4 minutes, or until the steak is almost cooked, shaking the basket once during cooking.
5. Stir in the mandarin oranges, and juice -mixture. Cook for 3 to 7 minutes more, or until the sauce is bubbling and the beef is tender and reaches at least 145°F on a meat thermometer.
6. Stir and serve over hot cooked cauliflower rice, if desired.

Nutrition:
Calories: 212
 Fat: 4g
 Saturated Fat: 1g
Protein: 19g
Carbohydrates: 28g
Sodium: 105mg
Fiber: 2g
Sugar: 22g

Simple Beef Sirloin Roast
Preparation Time: 10 minutes
Cooking Time: 50 minutes
Servings: 8
Ingredients:

- 2½ pounds sirloin roast
- Salt and ground black pepper, as required

Directions:
1. Rub the roast with salt and black pepper generously.
2. Insert the rotisserie rod through the roast.
3. Insert the rotisserie forks, one on each side of the rod to secure the rod to the chicken.

4. Arrange the drip pan in the bottom of Instant Vortex Plus Air Fryer Oven cooking chamber.
5. Select "Roast" and then adjust the temperature to 350 degrees F.
6. Set the timer for 50 minutes and press the "Start".
7. When the display shows "Add Food" press the red lever down and load the left side of the rod into the Vortex.
8. Now, slide the rod's left side into the groove along the metal bar so it doesn't move.
9. Then, close the door and touch "Rotate".
10. When cooking time is complete, press the red lever to release the rod.
11. Remove from the Vortex and place the roast onto a platter for about 10 minutes before slicing.
12. With a sharp knife, cut the roast into desired sized slices and serve.

Nutrition:
Calories 201
 Total Fat 8.8 g
Saturated Fat 3.1 g
Cholesterol 94 mg
Sodium 88 mg
Total Carbs 0 g
Fiber 0 g
Sugar 0 g
Protein 28.9 g

Fish

Old Bay Baked Cod
Preparation Time: 10 minutes
Cooking Time: 15 minutes
Servings: 4

Ingredients:
- 1 lb cod fillets
- 1/8 teaspoon dried basil
- 1/8 teaspoon old bay seasoning
- 1 tablespoon lemon juice
- 1 1/2 tablespoon mayonnaise
- 2 tablespoon butter, melted
- 1/4 cup parmesan cheese, grated

Directions:
1. In a bowl, mix together parmesan cheese, butter, mayonnaise, lemon juice, old bay seasoning, and basil.
2. Spread parmesan cheese mixture on top of fish fillets.
3. Place the cooking tray in the air fryer basket. Line air fryer basket with parchment paper.
4. Select Bake mode.
5. Set time to 15 minutes and temperature 350 F then press START.
6. The air fryer display will prompt you to ADD FOOD once the temperature is reached then place the fish fillet in the air fryer basket.
7. Serve and enjoy.

Nutrition:
Calories 211 Fat 11.8 g
Carbohydrates 1.9 g Sugar 0.4 g
Protein 25.1 g Cholesterol 83 mg

Baked Mayo Cod
Preparation Time: 10 minutes
Cooking Time: 10 minutes
Servings: 4
Ingredients:
- 4 cod fillets
- 1/2 cup almond flour

- 1 tablespoon parsley, chopped
- 1/2 teaspoon old bay seasoning
- 1/2 teaspoon lemon zest
- 1 tablespoon lemon juice
- 1/4 cup parmesan cheese, grated
- 1/4 cup onion, minced
- 2 tablespoon butter, melted
- 1/3 cup mayonnaise

Directions:

1. In a bowl, mix together mayonnaise, butter, onion, cheese, lemon juice, lemon zest, old bay seasoning, and parsley.
2. Spread mayonnaise mixture on top of fish fillets. Sprinkle with almond flour.
3. Place the cooking tray in the air fryer basket. Line air fryer basket with parchment paper.
4. Select Bake mode.
5. Set time to 10 minutes and temperature 400 F then press START.
6. The air fryer display will prompt you to ADD FOOD once the temperature is reached then place the fish fillet in the air fryer basket. Serve and enjoy.

Nutrition:
Calories 288 Fat 18.2 g Carbohydrates 6.8 g Sugar 1.8 g Protein 25.8 g Cholesterol 86 mg

Cajun Salmon Cakes

Preparation Time: 10 minutes
Cooking Time: 15 minutes
Servings: 4
Ingredients:

- 2 eggs, lightly beaten
- 12 oz can salmon, boneless & skinless
- 3/4 cup almond flour
- 2 1/2 teaspoon Cajun seasoning
- 1/2 onion, chopped
- 1/2 bell pepper, chopped
- 2 tablespoon mayonnaise
- Pepper
- Salt

Directions:

1. Add all ingredients into the mixing bowl and mix until well combined.
2. Make 8 equal shapes of patties from the mixture.
3. Place the cooking tray in the air fryer basket. Line air fryer basket with parchment paper.
4. Select Bake mode.
5. Set time to 10 minutes and temperature 375 F then press START.
6. The air fryer display will prompt you to ADD FOOD once the temperature is reached then add patties in the air fryer basket.
7. Broil patties for 5 minutes.
8. Serve and enjoy.

Nutrition:
Calories 212 Fat 9.6 g
Carbohydrates 5.5 g
Sugar 2.2 g Protein 22.9 g
Cholesterol 107 mg

Vegetable

Cheddar Cheese Broccoli

Preparation Time: 10 minutes
Cooking Time: 30 minutes

Servings: 6
Ingredients:

- 4 cups broccoli florets
- 1/4 cup ranch dressing
- 1/4 cup heavy whipping cream
- 1/2 cup cheddar cheese, shredded
- Pepper
- Salt

Directions:

1. Add all ingredients into the mixing bowl and mix until well coated.
2. Spread broccoli in baking dish.
3. Select Bake mode.
4. Set time to 30 minutes and temperature 375 F then press START.
5. The air fryer display will prompt you to ADD FOOD once the temperature is reached then place the baking dish in the air fryer basket.
6. Serve and enjoy.

Nutrition:
Calories 79
Fat 5.2 g
Carbohydrates 4.8 g
Sugar 1.4 g
Protein 4.3 g
Cholesterol 17 mg

Stuffed Bell Peppers

Preparation Time: 10 minutes
Cooking Time: 45 minutes
Servings: 4
Ingredients:

- 4 eggs
- 2 medium bell peppers, sliced in half and remove seeds
- 1/2 cup parmesan cheese, grated
- 1/2 cup mozzarella cheese, shredded
- 1/2 cup ricotta cheese
- 1/4 cup baby spinach
- 1/4 teaspoon dried parsley
- 1 teaspoon garlic powder

Directions:

1. Add three cheeses, parsley, garlic powder, and eggs in food processor and process until combined.
2. Pour egg mixture into each pepper half and top with baby spinach.
3. Place stuffed peppers in a baking dish. Cover dish with foil.
4. Select Bake mode.
5. Set time to 45 minutes and temperature 375 F then press START.
6. The air fryer display will prompt you to ADD FOOD once the temperature is reached then place the baking dish in the air fryer basket.
7. Serve and enjoy.

Nutrition:
Calories 232 Fat 13.9 g
Carbohydrates 8.2 g Sugar 3.6 g
Protein 20.2 g Cholesterol 196 mg

Baked Artichoke Spinach

Preparation Time: 10 minutes
Cooking Time: 20 minutes
Servings: 3
Ingredients:

- 6 oz artichoke hearts, chopped

- 4 oz cream cheese
- 1/8 teaspoon red pepper flakes
- 10 oz baby spinach
- 1 garlic clove, minced
- 1 tablespoon olive oil
- 2 oz brie cheese
- 1/3 cup black olives
- Pepper
- Salt

Directions:

1. Heat olive oil in a large pan over medium heat.
2. Add garlic and sauté for 1-2 minutes.
3. Add spinach, red pepper flakes, pepper, and salt and cook for 2-3 minutes or until spinach wilted.
4. Add cream cheese and cook until cheese is melted.
5. Add artichoke hearts and reduce heat. Cook for 3-5 minutes more.
6. Stir in olives. Transfer mixture to a baking dish and top with cheese. Select Bake mode.
7. Set time to 20 minutes and temperature 350 F then press START.
8. The air fryer display will prompt you to ADD FOOD once the temperature is reached then place the baking dish in the air fryer basket.

Nutrition:
Calories 302 Fat 25.2 g Carbohydrates 11.8 g Sugar 1.2 g Protein 11.5 g Cholesterol 60 mg

Delicious Zucchini Casserole

Preparation Time: 10 minutes
Cooking Time: 30 minutes
Servings: 6
Ingredients:

- 3 medium zucchini, sliced into 1/4-inch thick slices
- 1 tablespoon butter
- 2 tablespoon unsweetened almond milk
- 1/3 cup heavy cream
- 3 oz brie cheese
- 1/2 tablespoon Italian seasoning
- 1 cup Swiss gruyere cheese, shredded
- 2 garlic cloves, minced
- Pepper
- Salt

Directions:

1. Toss zucchini slices with salt and place into a colander and set aside for 45 minutes. Pat dry with a paper towel.
2. In a baking dish, arrange zucchini slices and season with pepper and salt.
3. Combine brie, garlic, butter, almond milk, and cream in a small saucepan and heat for few minutes or until cheese melts.
4. Pour cheese mixture over zucchini and sprinkle with shredded cheese.
5. Top with Italian seasoning.
6. Select Bake mode.
7. Set time to 30 minutes and temperature 400 F then press START.
8. The air fryer display will prompt you to ADD FOOD once the temperature is reached then place the baking dish in the air fryer basket.
9. Serve and enjoy.

Nutrition:
Calories 180
Fat 14.3 g
Carbohydrates 4 g
Sugar 1.9 g
Protein 9.1 g
Cholesterol 44 mg

Snacks

Butternut Squash Fries
Preparation time: 10 minutes
Cooking time: 18 minutes
Servings: 8
Ingredients:

- 1-pound butternut squash
- 1 teaspoon garlic powder
- 2 teaspoon sesame oil
- ½ teaspoon salt
- ½ teaspoon chili pepper

Directions:

1. Cut the butternut squash into strips and sprinkle with the garlic powder, sesame oil, salt, and chili pepper.
2. Massage the butternut squash slices using your fingertips.
3. Preheat the air fryer to 365 F.
4. Place the butternut squash fries in the air fryer and cook them for 18 minutes.
5. Stir frequently.
6. Allow to cool before serving.

Nutrition:
calories 32, fat 1.2, fiber 1.5, carbs 4.9, protein 0.8

Radish Chips
Preparation time: 10 minutes
Cooking time: 15 minutes
Servings: 7
Ingredients:

- 1 teaspoon ground red pepper
- 3 teaspoon olive oil
- ½ teaspoon ground black pepper
- 1 teaspoon salt
- 15 oz. daikon

Directions:

1. Combine the ground red pepper, olive oil, ground black pepper, and salt in a small bowl.
2. Whisk.
3. Slice the daikon into chips.
4. Preheat the air fryer to 375 F.
5. Brush daikon chips with the olive oil mixture.
6. Place the daikon chips in the air fryer rack.
7. Cook for 16 minutes.
8. Stir the daikon chips after 8 minutes of cooking.
9. Then chill the chips and serve.

Nutrition:
calories 30, fat 2,
fiber 1.3, carbs 2.7,
protein 1.3

Almond Pickles
Preparation time: 10 minutes
Cooking time: 10 minutes
Servings: 7
Ingredients:

- 12 oz. pickles

- 2 eggs
- 1 teaspoon salt
- 1 teaspoon ground black pepper
- ½ cup almond flour
- 1 tablespoon olive oil

Directions:

1. Slice the pickles.
2. Crack the eggs and whisk.
3. Combine the salt and ground black pepper. Stir the mixture.
4. Put the sliced pickles in the whisked egg mixture.
5. Sprinkle the sliced pickles with the salt mixture.
6. Dip the pickles into the egg mixture again.
7. Coat the pickles in the almond flour.
8. Preheat the air fryer to 400 F.
9. Grease the air fryer with olive oil.
10. Place the sliced pickles inside and cook for 10 minutes.
11. Serve warm.

Nutrition:
calories 53,
fat 4.4,
fiber 0.9,
carbs 1.8,
protein 2.2

Catfish Bites

Preparation time: 12 minutes
Cooking time: 16 minutes
Servings: 6
Ingredients:

- 1-pound catfish fillet
- 1 teaspoon minced garlic
- 1 large egg
- 2 oz chive stems, diced
- 1 tablespoon butter, melted
- 1 teaspoon turmeric
- 1 teaspoon ground thyme
- 1 teaspoon ground coriander
- ¼ teaspoon ground nutmeg
- 1 teaspoon flax seeds

Directions:

1. Cut the catfish fillet into 6 pieces.
2. Sprinkle the fish with the minced garlic. Stir.
3. Add diced chives, turmeric, ground thyme, ground coriander, ground nutmeg, and flax seeds.
4. Mix the catfish bites gently.
5. Preheat the air fryer to 360 F.
6. Coat the catfish bites with the melted butter then freeze them.
7. Put the catfish bites in the air fryer basket.
8. Cook the catfish bites for 16 minutes.

Nutrition:
calories 140,
fat 8.7,
fiber 0.5,
carbs 1.6,
protein 13.1

Dessert

Pecan Nutella

Preparation time: 20 minutes
Cooking time: 5 minutes
Servings: 4

Ingredients:

- 4 pecans, chopped
- 5 teaspoons butter, softened
- ½ teaspoon vanilla extract
- 1 tablespoon Splenda
- 1 teaspoon of cocoa powder

Directions:

1. Put all ingredients in the air fryer and stir gently.
2. Cook the mixture at 400F for 5 minutes.
3. Then transfer the mixture in the serving bowl and refrigerate for 15-20 minutes before serving.

Nutrition:
calories 157,
fat 14.8,
fiber 1.6,
carbs 5.3,
protein 1.6

Lemon Pie

Preparation Time: 10 minutes
Cooking time: 35 minutes
Servings: 6
Ingredients:

- 1 cup coconut flour
- ½ lemon, sliced
- ¼ cup heavy cream
- 2 eggs, beaten
- 2 tablespoons Erythritol
- 1 teaspoon baking powder
- Cooking spray

Directions:

1. Spray the air fryer basket with cooking spray.
2. Then line the bottom of the air fryer with lemon.
3. In the mixing bowl, mix coconut flour with heavy cream, eggs, Erythritol, and baking powder.
4. Pour the batter over the lemons and cook the pie at 365f for 35 minutes.

Nutrition:
calories 120, fat 5.3,
fiber 8.2,
carbs 14.4,
protein 4.7

Ricotta Cookies

Preparation Time: 15 minutes
Cooking time: 12 minutes
Servings: 6
Ingredients:

- 1 teaspoon vanilla extract
- 1 cup ricotta cheese
- 1 cup coconut flour
- 1 egg, beaten
- 2 tablespoons swerve

Directions:

1. Mix coconut flour with vanilla extract, ricotta cheese, egg, and swerve.
2. Knead the dough and make cookies.
3. Put the cookies in the air fryer and cook at 365F for 12 minutes.

Nutrition:
calories 150,
fat 6,
fiber 8,
carbs 15.6,
protein 8.3

Cream Cheese Pie

Preparation time: 15 minutes
Cooking time: 30 minutes
Servings: 6
Ingredients:

- 2 eggs, beaten
- 6 tablespoons almond flour
- ½ teaspoon vanilla extract
- 6 tablespoons cream cheese
- ½ teaspoon baking powder
- 1 teaspoon apple cider vinegar
- ½ teaspoon ground cinnamon
- 3 tablespoons Erythritol
- 1 tablespoon coconut oil, melted

Directions:
1. Brush the baking pan with coconut oil.
2. Then mix eggs with almond flour, vanilla extract, cream cheese, baking powder, apple cider vinegar, ground cinnamon, and Erythritol.
3. Blend the mixture until smooth and pour it in the baking pan.
4. Cook the pie in the air fryer at 350F for 30 minutes.
5. Then cool the cooked pie well.

Nutrition:
calories 120,
fat 10.6,
fiber 0.9,
carbs 2.3,
protein 4.1

Greece Style Cake
Preparation Time: 10 minutes
Cooking time: 30 minutes
Servings: 12
Ingredients:

- 6 eggs, beaten
- 1 teaspoon vanilla extract
- 1 teaspoon baking powder
- 2 cups almond flour
- 4 tablespoons Erythritol
- 1 cup Plain yogurt

Directions:
1. Mix all ingredients in the mixing bowl.
2. Then pour the mixture in the air fryer and flatten it gently.
3. Cook the cake at 350F for 30 minutes.

Nutrition:
calories 159,
fat 11.3,
fiber 2,
carbs 5.9,
protein 7.9

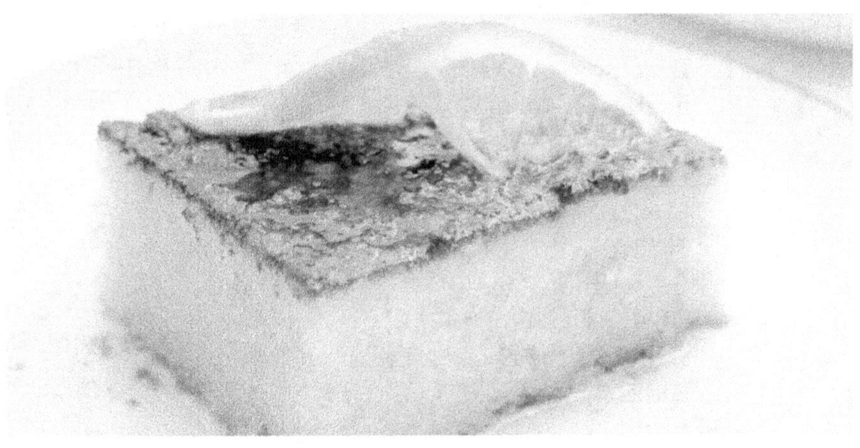

CHAPTER 14:

December

Lunch

Bacon Chicken Breast
Preparation time: 15 minutes
Cooking time: 16 minutes
Servings: 4
Ingredients:
- 1-pound chicken breast, skinless, boneless
- 4 oz. bacon, sliced
- 1 teaspoon paprika
- ¼ cup almond milk
- 1 teaspoon salt
- ½ teaspoon ground black pepper
- 1 teaspoon turmeric
- 1 tablespoon fresh lemon juice
- 2 tablespoon butter
- 1 teaspoon olive oil

Directions:
1. Beat the chicken breast lightly to flatten.
2. Then rub the chicken with the paprika, salt, ground black pepper, and turmeric.
3. Sprinkle the chicken with fresh lemon juice.
4. Then place the butter in the center of the chicken breast and roll it.
5. Wrap the chicken roll in the sliced bacon and sprinkle with the almond milk and olive oil.
6. Preheat the air fryer to 380 F.
7. Put the bacon chicken in the air fryer basket and cook it for 8 minutes.
8. Turn the chicken breast over and cook it for 8 minutes more.

Nutrition:
calories 383,
fat 25.4,
fiber 0.7,
carbs 2.2,
protein 35.1

Cheddar Chicken Drumsticks
Preparation time: 18 minutes
Cooking time: 13 minutes
Servings: 4
Ingredients:
- 1-pound chicken drumstick
- 6 oz. Cheddar cheese, sliced
- 1 teaspoon dried rosemary
- 1 teaspoon dried oregano
- ½ teaspoon salt
- ½ teaspoon chili flakes

Directions:
1. Sprinkle the chicken drumsticks with dried

2. Massage the drumsticks carefully and leave for 5 minutes to marinade.
3. Preheat the air fryer to 370 F.
4. Place the marinated chicken drumsticks in the air fryer tray and cook them for 10 minutes.
5. Turn the chicken drumsticks over and cover them with a layer of the sliced cheese.
6. Cook the chicken for 3 minutes more at the same temperature.
7. Then transfer the chicken drumsticks onto a large serving plate.
8. Serve the dish hot – the cheese should be melted.

Nutrition:
calories 226,
fat 9.8,
fiber 0.3,
carbs 1,
protein 16.4

Garlic Beef Steak

Preparation time: 15 minutes
Cooking time: 12 minutes
Servings: 4
Ingredients:

- 1 tablespoon butter
- 2 tablespoons fresh orange juice
- 1 teaspoon lime zest
- 1-pound beef steak
- 1 teaspoon ground ginger
- 1 teaspoon dried oregano
- 1 tablespoon cream
- ½ teaspoon minced garlic

Directions:

1. Combine the fresh orange juice, butter, lime zest, ground ginger, dried oregano, cream, and minced garlic together.
2. Combine the mixture well.
3. Then tenderize the steak gently.
4. Brush the beefsteak with the combined spice mix carefully and leave the steak for 7 minutes to marinade.
5. Preheat the air fryer to 360 F.
6. Put the marinated beef steak in the air fryer basket and cook the meat for 12 minutes. The beef should be well done.

Nutrition:
calories 245,
fat 10.2,
fiber 0.3,
carbs 1.7,
protein 34.6

Coriander Chicken

Preparation time: 20 minutes
Cooking time: 16 minutes
Servings: 4
Ingredients:

- 3 oz. fresh coriander root
- 1 teaspoon olive oil
- 3 tablespoon minced garlic
- ¼ lemon, sliced
- ½ teaspoon salt
- 1 teaspoon ground black pepper

- ½ teaspoon chili flakes
- 1 tablespoon dried parsley
- 1-pound chicken thighs

Directions:

1. Peel the fresh coriander and grate it.
2. Then combine the olive oil with the minced garlic, salt, ground black pepper, chili flakes, and dried parsley.
3. Combine the mixture and sprinkle over the chicken tights.
4. Add the sliced lemon and grated coriander root.
5. Mix the chicken thighs carefully and leave them to marinate for 10 minutes in the fridge.
6. Meanwhile, preheat the air fryer to 365 F.
7. Put the chicken in the air fryer basket tray.
8. Add all the remaining liquid from the chicken and cook for 15 minutes.
9. Turn the chicken over and cook it for 1 minute more.
10. Serve hot.

Nutrition:
calories 187, fat 11.4,
fiber 1, carbs 3.6,
protein 20

Air Frier Pork Ribs

Preparation time: 30 minutes
Cooking time: 30 minutes
Servings: 5
Ingredients:

- 1 tablespoon apple cider vinegar

- 1 teaspoon cayenne pepper
- 1 teaspoon minced garlic
- 1 teaspoon mustard
- 1 teaspoon chili flakes
- 16 oz. pork ribs
- 1 teaspoon sesame oil
- 1 teaspoon salt
- 1 tablespoon paprika

Directions:

1. Sprinkle the pork ribs with the cayenne pepper, apple cider vinegar, minced garlic, mustard, and chili flakes.
2. Add the sesame oil and salt.
3. Add paprika and mix into the pork ribs carefully.
4. Leave the ribs in the fridge for 20 minutes.
5. Preheat the air fryer to 360 F.
6. Transfer the pork ribs to the air fryer basket and cook them for 15 minutes.
7. Turn the pork ribs over and cook the meat for 15 minutes more.

Nutrition:
calories 265,
fat 17.4,
fiber 0.7,
carbs 1.4,
protein 24.5

Paprika Beef Tongue

Preparation time: 10 minutes
Cooking time: 20 minutes
Servings: 6
Ingredients:

- 1-pound beef tongue
- 1 teaspoon salt

- 1 teaspoon ground black pepper
- 1 teaspoon paprika
- 1 tablespoon butter
- 4 cup water

Directions:
1. Preheat the air fryer to 365 F.
2. Put the beef tongue in the air fryer basket tray and add water.
3. Sprinkle the mixture with salt, ground black pepper, and paprika.
4. Cook the beef tongue for 15 minutes.
5. Strain the water from the beef tongue.
6. Cut the beef tongue into strips.
7. Toss the butter in the air fryer basket tray and add the beef strips.
8. Cook the strips for 5 minutes at 360 F.
9. When the beef tongue is cooked transfer to a serving plate.

Nutrition:
calories 234, fat 18.8,
fiber 0.2,
carbs 0.4,
protein 14.7

Almond Salmon Pie

Preparation time: 20 minutes
Cooking time: 30 minutes
Servings: 8
Ingredients:

- ½ cup cream
- 1 ½ cup almond flour
- ½ teaspoon baking soda
- 1 tablespoon apple cider vinegar
- 1-pound salmon
- 1 tablespoon chives
- 1 teaspoon dried oregano
- 1 teaspoon dried dill
- 1 teaspoon butter
- 1 egg
- 1 teaspoon dried parsley
- 1 teaspoon ground paprika

Directions:
1. Crack the egg in a bowl and whisk it.
2. Add the cream and keep whisking it for 2 minutes more.
3. After this, add baking soda and apple cider vinegar.
4. Add almond flour and knead until you have a smooth and non-sticky dough.
5. Chop the salmon into tiny pieces.
6. Sprinkle the chopped salmon with the diced chives, dried oregano, dried dill, dried parsley, and ground paprika.
7. Mix well.
8. Cut the dough into 2 parts.
9. Cover the air fryer basket tray with parchment.
10. Put the first part of the dough in the air fryer basket tray and make the crust from it using your fingertips.
11. Then place the salmon filling.

12. Roll the second part of the dough with a rolling pin and cover the salmon filling.
13. Secure the pie edges.
14. Preheat the air fryer to 360 F.
15. Put the air fryer basket tray in the air fryer and cook for 15 minutes.
16. Then reduce to 355 F and cook the pie for 15 minutes more.
17. When the pie is cooked – remove it from the air fryer basket and allow to cool.

Nutrition:
calories 134,
fat 8.1,
fiber 1.1,
carbs 3.3,
protein 13.2

<u>Meat</u>

Seasoned Beef Roast
Preparation Time: 10 minutes
Cooking Time: 45 minutes
Servings: 10
Ingredients:

- 3 pounds beef top roast
- 1 tablespoon olive oil
- 2 tablespoons Montreal steak seasoning

Directions:

1. Coat the roast with oil and then rub with the seasoning generously.
2. With kitchen twines, tie the roast to keep it compact.
3. Arrange the roast onto the cooking tray.
4. Arrange the drip pan in the bottom of Instant Vortex Plus Air Fryer Oven cooking chamber.
5. Select "Air Fry" and then adjust the temperature to 360 degrees F.
6. Set the timer for 45 minutes and press the "Start".
7. When the display shows "Add Food" insert the cooking tray in the center position.
8. When the display shows "Turn Food" do nothing.
9. When cooking time is complete, remove the tray from Vortex and place the roast onto a platter for about 10 minutes before slicing.
10. With a sharp knife, cut the roast into desired sized slices and serve.

Nutrition:
Calories 269
Total Fat 9.9 g
Saturated Fat 3.4 g
Cholesterol 122 mg
Sodium 538 mg

Bacon Wrapped Filet Mignon
Preparation Time: 10 minutes
Cooking Time: 15 minutes
Servings: 2
Ingredients:

- 2 bacon slices
- 2 (4-ounce) filet mignon
- Salt and ground black pepper, as required
- Olive oil cooking spray

Directions:

1. Wrap 1 bacon slice around each filet mignon and secure with toothpicks.
2. Season the filets with the salt and black pepper lightly.

3. Arrange the filet mignon onto a coking rack and spray with cooking spray.
4. Arrange the drip pan in the bottom of Instant Vortex Plus Air Fryer Oven cooking chamber.
5. Select "Air Fry" and then adjust the temperature to 375 degrees F.
6. Set the timer for 15 minutes and press the "Start".
7. When the display shows "Add Food" insert the cooking rack in the center position.
8. When the display shows "Turn Food" turn the filets.
9. When cooking time is complete, remove the rack from Vortex and serve hot.

Nutrition:
Calories 360
Total Fat 19.6 g
 Saturated Fat 6.8 g
Cholesterol 108 mg
Sodium 737 mg
Total Carbs 0.4 g
 Fiber 0 g
Sugar 0 g
Protein 42.6 g

Beef Burgers

Preparation Time: 15 minutes
Cooking Time: 18 minutes
Servings: 4
Ingredients:
For Burgers:

- 1-pound ground beef
- ½ cup panko breadcrumbs
- ¼ cup onion, chopped finely
- 3 tablespoons Dijon mustard
- 3 teaspoons low-sodium soy sauce
- 2 teaspoons fresh rosemary, chopped finely
- Salt, to taste

For Topping:

- 2 tablespoons Dijon mustard
- 1 tablespoon brown sugar
- 1 teaspoon soy sauce
- 4 Gruyere cheese slices

Directions:

1. In a large bowl, add all the ingredients and mix until well combined.
2. Make 4 equal-sized patties from the mixture.
3. Arrange the patties onto a cooking tray.
4. Arrange the drip pan in the bottom of Instant Vortex Plus Air Fryer Oven cooking chamber.
5. Select "Air Fry" and then adjust the temperature to 370 degrees F.
6. Set the timer for 15 minutes and press the "Start".
7. When the display shows "Add Food" insert the cooking rack in the center position.
8. When the display shows "Turn Food" turn the burgers.
9. Meanwhile, for sauce: in a small bowl, add the mustard, brown sugar and soy sauce and mix well.
10. When cooking time is complete, remove the tray from Vortex and coat the burgers with the sauce.
11. Top each burger with 1 cheese slice.
12. Return the tray to the cooking chamber and select "Broil".
13. Set the timer for 3 minutes and press the "Start".

14. When cooking time is complete, remove the tray from Vortex and serve hot.

Nutrition:
Calories 402
Total Fat 18 g
Saturated Fat 8.5 g
Cholesterol 133mg
Sodium 651 mg
Total Carbs 6.3 g
Fiber 0.8 g
Sugar 3 g
Protein 44.4 g

Beef Jerky
Preparation Time: 15 minutes
Cooking Time: 3 hours
Servings: 4
Ingredients:

- 1½ pounds beef round, trimmed
- ½ cup Worcestershire sauce
- ½ cup low-sodium soy sauce
- 2 teaspoons honey
- 1 teaspoon liquid smoke
- 2 teaspoons onion powder
- ½ teaspoon red pepper flakes
- Ground black pepper, as required

Directions:

1. In a zip-top bag, place the beef and freeze for 1-2 hours to firm up.
2. Place the meat onto a cutting board and cut against the grain into 1/8-¼-inch strips.
3. In a large bowl, add the remaining ingredients and mix until well combined.
4. Add the steak slices and coat with the mixture generously.
5. Refrigerate to marinate for about 4-6 hours.
6. Remove the beef slices from bowl and with paper towels, pat dry them.
7. Divide the steak strips onto the cooking trays and arrange in an even layer.
8. Select "Dehydrate" and then adjust the temperature to 160 degrees F.
9. Set the timer for 3 hours and press the "Start".
10. When the display shows "Add Food" insert 1 tray in the top position and another in the center position.
11. After 1½ hours, switch the position of cooking trays.
12. Meanwhile, in a small pan, add the remaining ingredients over medium heat and cook for about 10 minutes, stirring occasionally.
13. When cooking time is complete, remove the trays from Vortex.

Nutrition:
Calories 372 Total Fat 10.7 g
 Saturated Fat 4 g Cholesterol 152 mg
Sodium 2000 mg
Total Carbs 12 g Fiber 0.2 g
Sugar 11.3 g Protein 53.8 g

Dinner

Roasted Air Fryer Savory Carrots
Basic Recipe
Preparation Time: 10 minutes
Cooking Time: 20 minutes
Servings: 4
Ingredients:

- 1 lb. medium sized carrots (washed and peeled)
- ¼ cup grated parmesan cheese

- Fresh chopped parsley (optional)
- 2 tablespoon olive oil
- ½ tsp. paprika
- ½ tsp. garlic powder
- Salt and pepper (to taste)

Directions:

1. Place peeled and chopped carrots in a large bowl, add olive oil, and toss in garlic powder and paprika
2. Put the carrot mix in an air fryer basket and cook on 380ºF for 10 minutes, shake and cook for another 10 minutes in the same heat.
3. Once the carrot is done, use parsley and parmesan cheese as topping and add pepper and salt to taste.

Nutrition:
Calories 119
Fat 6g
Protein 1g
Carbs 17g

Broccoli Creamy Casserole
Basic Recipe
Preparation Time: 5 minutes
Cooking Time: 30 minutes
Servings: 4
Ingredients:

- 1 cup diced ham
- 1 (14-ounce) bags frozen broccoli
- 4 ounces' cream cheese, softened
- ½ cup plain full-fat greek yogurt
- ¼ cup mayonnaise
- ½ teaspoon garlic salt
- ½ teaspoon onion powder
- ½ teaspoon dried basil
- ½ teaspoon smoked paprika
- ¼ teaspoon rosemary

- ¼ teaspoon thyme
- ½ cup shredded cheese
- ½ cup crushed pork rinds

Directions:

1. Preheat air fryer to 350-degrees F. Spray a 6-inch soufflé dish with non-stick cooking spray; set aside.
2. Mix the ham, broccoli, cream cheese, yoghurt, mayonnaise, garlic salt, onion powder, basil, smoked paprika, rosemary and thyme in a large bowl.
3. Pour the batter into a oiled pan and cover the pan with grated cheese and shredded rinds. Bake it for 25 minutes or until the pan is golden and bubbly.

Nutrition:
Calories 273,
Fat 17.4g,
Carbs 9.7g
Protein 17.4g

Chicken, Feta, and Olive Casserole
Basic Recipe
Preparation Time: 5 minutes
Cooking Time: 30 minutes
Servings: 4
Ingredients:
Chicken Casserole

- 1½ pounds boneless chicken thighs
- Salt and pepper, to taste
- 2 tablespoons butter
- 3 ounces pesto
- 1¼ cups coconut cream
- 3 ounces' green olives
- 5 ounces diced feta cheese
- 1 clove garlic, finely chopped

For Serving:

- 5 ounces leafy greens
- 4 tablespoons coconut oil
- Salt and pepper, to taste

Directions:

1. Preheat air fryer to 350-degrees F. Spray a 6-inch soufflé dish with non-stick cooking spray; set aside.
2. Put the butter in a large saucepan. Heat the pan until the butter is melt, then sauté the chicken pieces until golden.
3. Combine pesto and cream in a container to make the sauce. Put the chicken, olives, feta, and garlic and pesto sauce in a saucepan.
4. Mix well and Bake it for 30 minutes in air fryer or until the edges are hot and brown

Nutrition:

Calories 643
Fat 56.7g
Carbs: 5.7g
Protein 28.5g

Sesame-Crusted Cod with Cauliflower

Basic Recipe
Preparation Time: 5 minutes
Cooking Time: 20 minutes
Servings: 4
Ingredients:

- 4 (5 ounce) cod fillets
- Salt and ground black pepper to taste
- 3 tablespoons butter, melted
- 2 tablespoons sesame seeds
- Coconut oil
- 1 small head cauliflower
- 3 cloves garlic, thinly sliced
- 1 lemon, cut into wedges

Directions:

1. Gently grease the air fryer basket with coconut oil and preheat to 400 degrees F.
2. Defrost fish if frozen; dry with kitchen paper, and lightly Season it with salt and pepper.
3. At the same time mix butter and sesame seeds in a bowl. Keep aside 2 tablespoons of the butter and sesame batter for the fish. Toss cauliflower and garlic with remaining butter batter and put into the air fryer basket.
4. Cook cauliflower in the preheated air fryer in parts, if required, until just cooked, tossing once, about 10 minutes Remove and keep warm while cooking fish.
5. Grease fish with 1/2 of the remaining butter batter. Put fillets in air fryer basket. Cook 4 minutes; shift fish. Grease with remaining butter batter. Cook 5 to 6 minutes more or until fish starts to flake when tested with a fork. Serve with cauliflower and lemon wedges.

Nutrition:

Calories 181
Fat 14.7g
Carbs 7.2g
Protein 7g

Stevia -Cajun Chicken Thighs

Basic Recipe
Preparation Time: 10 minutes
Cooking Time: 25 minutes
Servings: 4
Ingredients:

- 1 ½ pounds skinless, boneless chicken thighs

- ¼ cup coconut flour
- ⅓cup almond flour
- 2 ½ teaspoons cajun seasoning
- ½ teaspoon garlic powder
- ½ teaspoon stevia powder
- ¼ teaspoon ground paprika
- ⅛ teaspoon cayenne pepper
- ¼ teaspoon salt

Directions:

1. Mix coconut flour, almond flour, Cajun spice, garlic powder, salt, stevia powder, paprika and cayenne pepper in a dish. The thighs distribute the flour mixture. Remove extra flour
2. Preheat a deep fryer to 175 °C (360 degrees F). Place the chicken legs in the frying basket and let them done within 15 minutes Turn the legs over and done until the chicken legs in the middle are it is no longer pink and the juice comes out clearly for about 10 minutes longer.
3. A quick reading thermometer in the middle should show at least 74 ° C (165 ° F). Take the chicken legs out of the deep fryer and sprinkle the lemon juice over each leg.

Nutrition:
Calories 121 Fat 9.1g
Carbs 3.3g Protein 7.2g

Bang-Bang chicken
Basic Recipe
Preparation Time: 10 minutes
Cooking Time: 15 minutes
Servings: 4
Ingredients:

- 1 cup Greek Yogurt
- ½ cup Sweet chili sauce
- 2 tablespoons hot sauce
- ⅓Cup Coconut flour
- 1-pound Chicken breast tenderloins cut into bite-size pieces
- 1 ½ cups Panko bread crumbs
- 2 Green onions, chopped

Directions:

1. Whisk Greek yogurt, sweet chili sauce and hot sauce in a large container. Set the 3/4 cup of the batter aside with a spoon and put the coconut flour in a plastic bag with a large seal.
2. Add the chicken, close the bag, and mix well to cover. Place the coated chicken pieces with the yoghurt mixture in the large container and stir.
3. Place the panko breadcrumbs in other big plastic bag with a zipper. Work in batches, place chicken pieces in panko, close and mixed well covered.
4. Preheat an air fryer to 200 ° C. Place as many pieces of chicken as possible in the basket without overfilling them, Cook in an air fryer for at least 10 minutes
5. Turn around and cook another 5 minutes repetition with the rest of the chicken Transfer the fried chicken to a large container and put the reaming sauce over it.
6. Sprinkle with spring onions and cover and stir. Serve immediately.

Nutrition:
Calories 303 Fat 15.3g
Carbs 10.9g Protein 17.1g

Fish

Blackened Tilapia
Preparation Time: 10 minutes
Cooking Time: 14 minutes
Servings: 3
Ingredients:

- 3 tilapia fillets
- 1 tablespoon dried parsley flakes
- 1/4 teaspoon cayenne pepper
- 1 teaspoon garlic powder
- 1 teaspoon onion powder
- 2 1/2 tablespoon paprika
- 1/2 teaspoon pepper
- 1 teaspoon salt

Directions:

1. In a small bowl, mix together paprika, pepper, onion powder, garlic powder, cayenne, parsley, pepper, and salt.
2. Spray fish fillets with cooking spray.
3. Rub the paprika mixture on both sides of fish fillets.
4. Place the cooking tray in the air fryer basket. Line air fryer basket with parchment paper.
5. Select Bake mode.
6. Set time to 14 minutes and temperature 400 F then press START.
7. The air fryer display will prompt you to ADD FOOD once the temperature is reached then place the fish fillet in the air fryer basket.
8. Serve and enjoy.

Nutrition:
Calories 117
Fat 1.8 g
Carbohydrates 4.9 g
Sugar 1.1 g
Protein 22.2 g
Cholesterol 55 mg

Garlic Butter Baked Shrimp
Preparation Time: 10 minutes
Cooking Time: 8 minutes
Servings: 4
Ingredients:

- 1 1/2 lbs shrimp, peeled & deveined
- 1/4 cup parmesan cheese, grated
- 1/2 teaspoon paprika
- 1 teaspoon garlic powder
- 1/4 teaspoon pepper
- 1/4 cup butter, melted
- 1 teaspoon kosher salt

Directions:

1. Add shrimp and remaining ingredients into the large bowl and toss well.
2. Place the cooking tray in the air fryer basket. Line air fryer basket with parchment paper.
3. Select Bake mode.
4. Set time to 8 minutes and temperature 400 F then press START.
5. The air fryer display will prompt you to ADD FOOD once the temperature is reached then add shrimp in the air fryer basket.
6. Serve and enjoy.

Nutrition:
Calories 354 Fat 17.5 g
Carbohydrates 3.8 g
Sugar 0.2 g
Protein 43.7 g
Cholesterol 399 mg

Cajun Catfish Fillets

Preparation Time: 10 minutes
Cooking Time: 25 minutes
Servings: 2
Ingredients:

- 2 catfish fillets
- 1/2 tablespoon olive oil
- 1/2 teaspoon red pepper flakes, crushed
- 1/2 teaspoon oregano
- 1/2 teaspoon paprika
- 1/2 teaspoon cayenne pepper
- 1/2 teaspoon onion powder
- 1/2 teaspoon garlic powder
- Pepper
- Salt

Directions:

1. In a small bowl, mix together garlic powder, onion powder, cayenne pepper, paprika, oregano, red pepper flakes, pepper, and salt.
2. Brush fish fillets with olive oil and rub with spice mixture.
3. Place the cooking tray in the air fryer basket. Line air fryer basket with parchment paper.
4. Select Bake mode.
5. Set time to 25 minutes and temperature 350 F then press START.
6. The air fryer display will prompt you to ADD FOOD once the temperature is reached then place fish fillets in the air fryer basket.
7. Serve and enjoy.

Nutrition:
Calories 256 Fat 15.9 g Carbohydrates 2.1 g Sugar 0.6 g Protein 25.3 g Cholesterol 75 mg

Vegetable

Cheesy Baked Zoodle

Preparation Time: 10 minutes
Cooking Time: 35 minutes
Servings: 4
Ingredients:

- 2 medium zucchini, spiralized
- 2 tablespoon butter
- 1 teaspoon fresh thyme, chopped
- 1 small onion, sliced
- 1 cup Fontina cheese, grated
- 2 teaspoon Worcestershire sauce
- 1/4 cup vegetable broth
- Pepper
- Salt

Directions:

1. Melt butter in a pan over medium heat.
2. Add the onion in a pan and sauté for a few minutes.
3. Add thyme, Worcestershire sauce, pepper, and salt. Stir for minutes.
4. Add broth in the pan and cook onions for 10 minutes.
5. In a large bowl, combine together zucchini noodles and onion mixture and pour into the greased baking dish.
6. Top with grated cheese.
7. Select Bake mode.
8. Set time to 25 minutes and temperature 400 F then press START.
9. The air fryer display will prompt you to ADD FOOD once the temperature is reached then place the baking dish in the air fryer basket.

10. Garnish with thyme and serve.

Nutrition:

Calories 184 Fat 14.5 g

Carbohydrates 6.1 g Sugar 3.4 g

Protein 8.7 g Cholesterol 47 mg

Parmesan Squash Casserole

Preparation Time: 10 minutes

Cooking Time: 45 minutes

Servings: 4

Ingredients:

- 4 medium squash, cut into slices
- 1/4 cup parmesan cheese, shredded
- 3/4 stick butter, cut into cubes
- 1 medium onion, sliced
- Pepper
- Salt

Directions:

1. Layer slices squash, onion, butter, pepper, and salt. Sprinkle with shredded parmesan cheese in a baking dish.
2. Cover dish with foil.
3. Select Bake mode.
4. Set time to 45 minutes and temperature 350 F then press START.
5. The air fryer display will prompt you to ADD FOOD once the temperature is reached then place the baking dish in the air fryer basket.
6. Serve and enjoy.

Nutrition:

Calories 241 Fat 20.7 g

Carbohydrates 9.7 g Sugar 4.6 g

Protein 7.5 g Cholesterol 56 mg

Pecan Green Bean Casserole

Preparation Time: 10 minutes

Cooking Time: 20 minutes

Servings: 4

Ingredients:

- 1 lb green beans, trimmed and cut into pieces
- 1/4 cup olive oil
- 2 oz pecans, crushed
- 1 small onion, chopped
- 2 tablespoon lemon zest
- 1/4 cup parmesan cheese, shredded

Directions:

1. Add all ingredients into the mixing bowl and toss well.
2. Spread green bean mixture into the baking dish.
3. Select Bake mode.
4. Set time to 20 minutes and temperature 400 F then press START.
5. The air fryer display will prompt you to ADD FOOD once the temperature is reached then place the baking dish in the air fryer basket.
6. Serve and enjoy.

Nutrition:

Calories 297

Fat 26 g

Carbohydrates 12.9 g

Sugar 3 g

Protein 8.5 g

Cholesterol 10 mg

Delicious Spaghetti Squash

Preparation Time: 10 minutes
Cooking Time: 10 minutes
Servings: 4
Ingredients:

- 2 cups spaghetti squash, cooked and drained
- 4 oz mozzarella cheese, cubed
- 1/4 cup basil pesto
- 1/2 cup ricotta cheese
- 1 tablespoon olive oil
- Pepper
- Salt

Directions:

1. In a bowl, combine together olive oil and squash. Season with pepper and salt.
2. Spread squash mixture in a baking dish.
3. Spread mozzarella cheese and ricotta cheese on top.
4. Select Bake mode.
5. Set time to 10 minutes and temperature 375 F then press START.
6. The air fryer display will prompt you to ADD FOOD once the temperature is reached then place the baking dish in the air fryer basket.
7. Drizzle with basil pesto and serve.

Nutrition:
Calories 169 Fat 11.3 g
Carbohydrates 6.1 g Sugar 0.1 g
Protein 11.9 g Cholesterol 25 mg

Cauliflower Casserole

Preparation Time: 10 minutes
Cooking Time: 15 minutes
Servings: 6
Ingredients:

- 1 cauliflower head, cut into florets and boil
- 1 cup cheddar cheese, shredded
- 1 cup mozzarella cheese, shredded
- 2 oz cream cheese
- 1 cup heavy cream
- 1/2 teaspoon pepper
- 1/2 teaspoon salt

Directions:

1. Add cream in a small saucepan and bring to simmer, stir well. Add cream cheese and stir until thickens.
2. Remove from heat and add 1 cup shredded cheddar cheese and seasoning and stir well.
3. Place boiled cauliflower florets into the greased baking dish. Pour saucepan mixture over cauliflower florets. Sprinkle mozzarella cheese over the cauliflower mixture. Select Bake mode. Set time to 15 minutes and temperature 375 F then press START. The air fryer display will prompt you to ADD FOOD once the temperature is reached then place the baking dish in the air fryer basket. Serve and enjoy.

Nutrition:
Calories 203 Fat 17.8 g Carbohydrates 3.7 g
Sugar 1.2 g Protein 8 g Cholesterol 60 mg

Basil Eggplant Casserole

Preparation Time: 10 minutes
Cooking Time: 35 minutes
Servings: 6
Ingredients:

- 1 eggplant, sliced
- 3 zucchini, sliced
- 4 tablespoon basil, chopped
- 1 tablespoon olive oil
- 3 garlic cloves, minced
- 3 oz mozzarella cheese, grated
- 1/4 cup parsley, chopped
- 1/4 teaspoon pepper
- 1/4 teaspoon salt

Directions:

1. Add all ingredients into the large bowl and toss well to combine.
2. Pour eggplant mixture into the greased baking dish.
3. Select Bake mode.
4. Set time to 35 minutes and temperature 350 F then press START.
5. The air fryer display will prompt you to ADD FOOD once the temperature is reached then place the baking dish in the air fryer basket.
6. Serve and enjoy.

Nutrition:
Calories 104 Fat 5.3 g
Carbohydrates 10.2 g
Sugar 4.8 g
Protein 6.4 g
Cholesterol 8 mg

Brussels Sprouts and Broccoli

Preparation Time: 10 minutes

Cooking Time: 30 minutes
Servings: 6
Ingredients:

- 1 lb broccoli, cut into florets
- 1 lb Brussels sprouts, cut ends
- 1 teaspoon paprika
- 1/2 onion, chopped
- 1 teaspoon garlic powder
- 1/2 teaspoon pepper
- 3 tablespoon olive oil
- 3/4 teaspoon salt

Directions:

1. Add all ingredients into the mixing bowl and toss well.
2. The spread vegetable mixture in a baking dish.
3. Select Bake mode.
4. Set time to 30 minutes and temperature 400 F then press START.
5. The air fryer display will prompt you to ADD FOOD once the temperature is reached then place the baking dish in the air fryer basket.
6. Serve and enjoy.

Nutrition:
Calories 122
Fat 7.3 g
Carbohydrates 11.9 g
Sugar 2.2 g
Protein 5.5 g
Cholesterol 0 mg

Snacks

Almond Onion Squares

Preparation time: 15 minutes
Cooking time: 8 minutes

Servings: 8
Ingredients:

- 2 white onions
- 1 cup almond flour
- 1 teaspoon baking powder
- ¼ tablespoon salt
- 1 cup heavy cream
- 1 teaspoon paprika
- 1 teaspoon sesame oil

Directions:

1. Peel the onions and cut them into medium squares.
2. Combine the almond flour, baking powder, salt, and paprika in a large bowl.
3. Stir the dried mixture with a fork.
4. Put the onion squares in the heavy cream and coat well.
5. Sprinkle the onion squares with the dried spice mixture on each side.
6. Drizzle the onion squares with the sesame oil.
7. Preheat the air fryer to 360 F.
8. Put the onion squares in the air fryer and cook for 8 minutes.

Nutrition:
calories 89,
fat 7.9,
fiber 1.1,
carbs 4.2,
protein 1.4

Parmesan Beans

Preparation time: 12 minutes
Cooking time: 5 minutes
Servings: 7
Ingredients:

- 14 oz. green beans
- 5 oz. Parmesan, shredded
- 1 egg
- 2 tablespoon coconut flakes
- 1 teaspoon dried oregano
- ½ teaspoon ground paprika
- 1 teaspoon butter

Directions:

1. Wash the green beans.
2. Crack the egg in a bowl and whisk it.
3. Preheat the air fryer to 400 F.
4. Place the green beans in the whisked egg.
5. Sprinkle the green beans with the coconut flakes, dried oregano, and ground paprika.
6. Then add the shredded cheese and stir carefully.
7. Put the butter in the air fryer basket and melt it.
8. Add the green beans.
9. Cook for 5 minutes.
10. Stir the green beans and separate it into 7 servings.

Nutrition:
calories 103,
fat 6.1,
fiber 2.2,
carbs 5.3,
protein 8.4

Cod Fries

Preparation time: 10 minutes
Cooking time: 6 minutes
Servings: 6
Ingredients:

- 1-pound cod fillet
- 2 large eggs
- 1 tablespoon coconut oil
- ½ teaspoon salt
- 1 teaspoon ground black pepper
- 1 teaspoon turmeric
- 1 teaspoon paprika

Directions:

1. Cut the cod fillet into 6 parts (fries size).
2. Crack the egg in a bowl and whisk it.
3. Add the salt, ground black pepper, turmeric, and paprika.
4. Stir.
5. Dip the cod fillets in the egg mixture.
6. Preheat the air fryer to 360 F.
7. Top the cod fillets with the coconut oil and put them in the air fryer rack.
8. Cook the dish for 6 minutes stirring after 4 minutes.
9. Remove the cooked fish fries from the air fryer.
10. Serve the dish with keto sauce.

Nutrition:
calories 107,
fat 4.7,
fiber 0.3,
carbs 0.8,
protein 15.7

Bacon Brussels Sprouts

Preparation time: 15 minutes
Cooking time: 12 minutes
Servings: 6
Ingredients:

- 6 oz. bacon, sliced
- 16 oz. Brussel sprouts
- ½ teaspoon salt
- 2 teaspoon coconut flakes
- ¼ teaspoon ground red pepper
- 1 teaspoon apple cider vinegar
- 1 tablespoon olive oil

Directions:

1. Wash Brussels sprouts.
2. Coat the bacon with salt, coconut flakes, and ground red pepper.
3. Drizzle the Brussel sprouts with the apple cider vinegar and olive oil.
4. Wrap Brussels sprouts in the sliced bacon. Secure with toothpicks if preffered.
5. Preheat the air fryer to 365 F.
6. Put wrapped Brussel sprouts in the air fryer and cook for 12 minutes.

Nutrition:
calories 208,
fat 14.6,
fiber 2.9,
carbs 7.4,
protein 13.1

Dessert

Pecan Cobbler

Preparation time: 15 minutes
Cooking time: 30 minutes
Servings: 4
Ingredients:

- ¼ cup coconut cream
- 1 egg, beaten
- ½ cup coconut flour
- 1 teaspoon vanilla extract
- 2 tablespoons coconut oil, softened
- 3 pecans, chopped

Directions:

1. Mix coconut oil with pecans and put the mixture in the air fryer. Flatten the mixture gently.
2. In the mixing bowl, mix coconut cream with egg, coconut flour, and vanilla extract.
3. Put the mixture over the pecans, flatten it gently and cook at 350F for 30 minutes.
4. Cool the cooked meal and transfer in the plates.

Nutrition:
calories 245,
fat 20.5,
fiber 7.5,
carbs 12.5,
protein 4.8

Cocoa Pudding

Preparation Time: 10 minutes
Cooking time: 20 minutes
Servings: 8
Ingredients:

- 2 cups ricotta cheese
- 2 tablespoons coconut flour
- 3 tablespoons Splenda
- 3 eggs, beaten
- 1 tablespoon vanilla extract
- ½ cup coconut cream
- 1 tablespoon cocoa powder

Directions:

1. Whisk the coconut cream with cocoa powder.
2. Then add eggs, Splenda, ricotta cheese, and coconut flour.
3. Mix the mixture until smooth and pour in the air fryer.
4. Cook the pudding at 350F for 20 minutes. Stir the pudding every 5 minutes during cooking.

Nutrition:
calories 180,
fat 10.4,
fiber 1.3,
carbs 10.5,
protein 9.9

Lemon Biscotti

Preparation time: 15 minutes
Cooking time: 40 minutes
Servings: 6
Ingredients:

- 2 oz almonds, chopped
- 2 tablespoons coconut oil
- 2 eggs, beaten
- 1 teaspoon vanilla extract
- 1 cup coconut flour
- 1 teaspoon lemon zest, grated
- ½ teaspoon baking powder
- 1 teaspoon lemon juice
- ¼ cup coconut cream
- 1 teaspoon sesame oil
- 3 tablespoons Erythritol

Directions:
1. Mix all ingredients in the mixing bowl.
2. Then knead the dough and put in the air fryer basket.
3. Cook the dough for 38 minutes at 375F.
4. Then slice the dough into biscotti and cook at 400F for 2 minutes more.

Nutrition:
calories 227, fat 15.9,
fiber 9.4, carbs 16.4,
protein 6.8

Sweet Carambola Chips

Preparation time: 10 minutes
Cooking time: 50 minutes
Servings: 6
Ingredients:
- 10 oz carambola, sliced
- 1 teaspoon coconut oil, melted
- 1 tablespoon Erythritol

Directions:
1. Mix carambola with coconut oil and Erythritol.
2. Then put it in the air fryer and cook at 340F for 50 minutes. Shake the carambola slices every 5 minutes.

Nutrition:
calories 21, fat 0.9,
fiber 1.3, carbs 3.2, protein 0.5

Chia Pie

Preparation Time: 10 minutes
Cooking time: 30 minutes
Servings: 8
Ingredients:
- 1 cup almond flour
- 2 tablespoons chia seeds
- 4 eggs, beaten
- 4 tablespoons Erythritol
- 1 teaspoon vanilla extract
- 2 tablespoons coconut oil, melted

Directions:
1. Brush the air fryer basket with coconut oil.
2. Then mix almond flour with chia seeds, eggs, vanilla extract, and Erythritol.
3. Put the mixture in the air fryer basket, flatten it in the shape of the pie and cook at 365F for 30 minutes.

Nutrition:
calories 164,
fat 13.3,
fiber 2.7,
carbs 4.7,
protein 6.4

Conclusion

Thank you for purchasing this book. The book was a result of my sincere endeavor to offer you fantastic air fryer recipes. It can help you indulge in healthy eating by not having to bury the desire to enjoy deep-fried foods. I have been creating various air fryer recipes that are easy to cook for a long time, and this cookbook consists of various types of air fry recipes for every day.

All the recipes are quick and suit healthy living. The delicious air fryer recipes in this book are categorized by breakfast, lunch, dinner, appetizers, seafood, side dishes, snacks, and desserts. Tried and tested recipes were used in this book to make sure that the foods taste good exactly the way how you cook with a conventional appliance for deep frying. You will get the crispness, the fried aroma, the browning, taste, and whatnot.

My collection of air fryer recipes would be the biggest inspiration for you to switch to a healthy version of fried foods. This book will be a detailed guide on how to cook some of your favorite meals without using oil that will not just be healthy but also packed with texture and rich flavor.

You can forget about the menace of oil, which creates havoc to your body and one of the main culprits to make people obese. I have taken special care to include recipes that are simple, tasty, and easy to Prepare. I wish you all a happy, healthy living and a new style of cooking!

Though, people who wish to have a balanced personal and office life, sometimes find it impossible to spend quality time with family by cooking a good healthy meal. An air fryer and a cookbook with recipes can help you make it a thing of the past. The cookbook, loaded with a rich and satisfying collection of recipes, will let you enjoy warm accolades from everyone who tastes your air fryer food.

While an air fryer seems like a specialized and expensive kitchen appliance, it is not the one that would sit on your kitchen countertop forever. In addition to cooking healthy fried food, you can also grill, roast, bake, stir fry and steam in this delightful appliance. I'm sure you would end up using it every day to eat healthily.

If you don't have an air fryer, purchase one now or if you already have one, but you rarely use it, check out my simple yet delectable recipe collection to get started. What more could you ask for? Now is the time to change the way you cook. With an air fryer, you can recreate and continue enjoying that deep-fried food you loved but may have given up just because it is deep-fried in excess oil.

Index

C

D

E

R

S

www.ingramcontent.com/pod-product-compliance
Lightning Source LLC
Chambersburg PA
CBHW081950260726
48657CB00009BA/2519